Britain's Crimea Nurses

Britain's Crimea Nurses

Two Accounts of the Women Who Tended the Wounded Soldiers of the Crimean War, 1853-56

Eastern Hospitals and English Nurses
(Volumes 1 & 2 in one special edition)
A Lady Volunteer

Memories of the Crimea
Sister Mary Aloysius

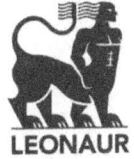

Britain's Crimea Nurses
Two Accounts of the Women Who Tended the Wounded Soldiers of the Crimean War, 1853-56
Eastern Hospitals and English Nurses
(Volumes 1 & 2 in one special edition)
by A Lady Volunteer
and
Memories of the Crimea
by Sister Mary Aloysius

FIRST EDITION IN THIS FORM

First published under the titles
Eastern Hospitals and English Nurses Volumes 1 and 2
and
Memories of the Crimea

Leonaur is an imprint of Oakpast Ltd
Copyright in this form © 2025 Oakpast Ltd

ISBN: 978-1-917666-52-7 (hardcover)
ISBN: 978-1-917666-53-4 (softcover)

http://www.leonaur.com

Publisher's Notes

The views expressed in this book are not necessarily those of the publisher.

Contents

Eastern Hospitals and English Nurses   7
Memories of the Crimea   221

Eastern Hospitals and English Nurses

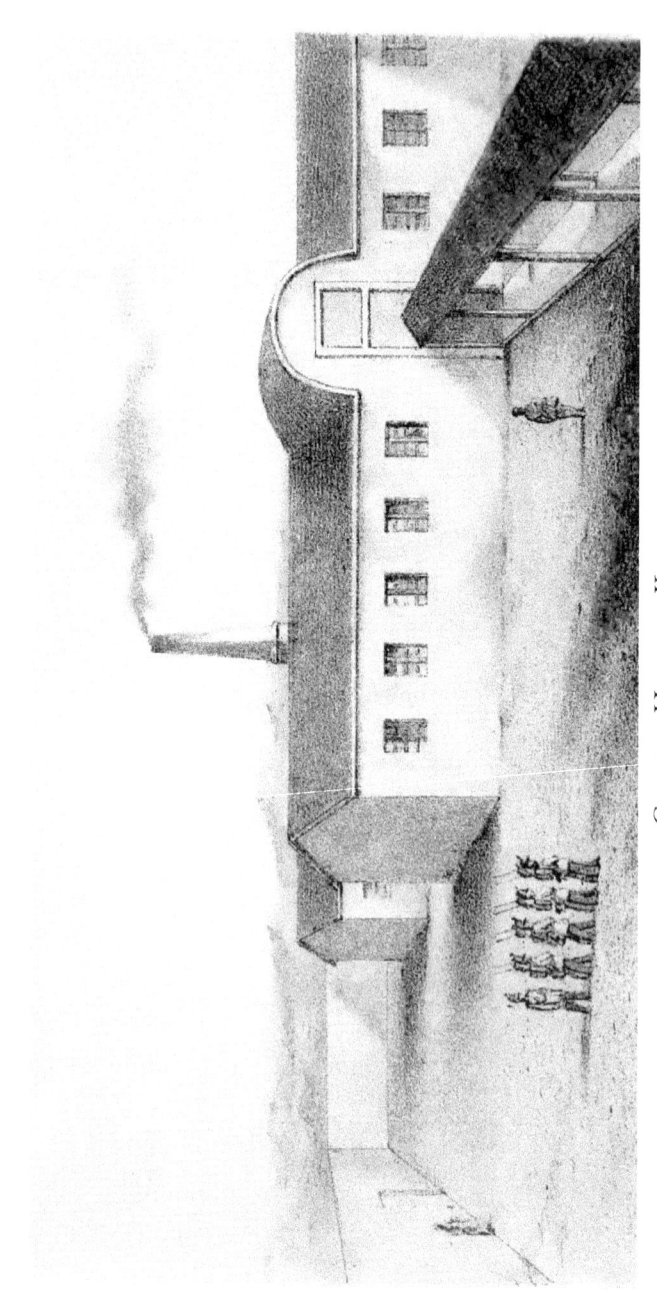

General Hospital, Koulali

Contents

Preface	13
News of the Battle of the Alma	15
Passage down the Rhone to Valence	20
Continued Delay at Therapia	26
The General Hospital, Scutari	36
Koulali	49
Arrival of Irish Soldiers at the Hospital	52
Unwearied Zeal of the Sisters of Mercy	60
The Plague of Rats	66
The Old Age of Sickness	74
Russian Prisoners	82
A Terrible Cholera Case	92
The Starving System	99
The General Hospital at Koulali	103
Heartbreaking Work	109
Shopping at Pera	114
Soeur Bernardine	122
Difficulties and Impossibilities	128

Cooks Sent Out by Government	135
Affection of the Irish Soldiers for Their Nuns	141
The Free Gift Store	145
A Fearful Accident	148
The Crescent and the Cross	156
The Nuns' Careful Nursing	165
Frequent Fires in Constantinople	170
The Religious Spirit in the British Army	174
Regimental and Camp Hospitals	177
Departure of the Sisters for Balaclava	182
The Bazaars of Stamboul	186
Visions of the Past	194
Traces of the Knights of Malta	203
Accounts from Balaclava	214

To those of
The British Army
Who displayed their heroism
Not only on the battlefield,
But in the
Patient endurance of suffering, privation, and neglect,
In the wards of Eastern hospitals,
This work
Is dedicated.

Preface

The deep interest taken by the People of England in all that relates to their army engaged in the Crimean campaign, has been met by innumerable details of the valour of the soldiers on the field, and of their patient endurance amidst the hardships of the siege; but of the heroism displayed by those who suffered in the obscurity of the Hospital Ward, there has been as yet but slight mention made. For this reason, one of the band of Englishwomen who went out, and assisted in alleviating the sufferings of the sick and wounded soldiers, ventures on her return to lay before her countrymen some account of the sufferings and the uncomplaining patience of those brave men, and also of the gradual improvements that were subsequently made in the hospitals.

And, knowing that very many persons took a deep interest in the proceedings of the nurses, the writer has felt encouraged to add a narrative of their domestic life, and of the perplexities which often beset them, as well as of the pleasing and amusing incidents which occasionally varied the scene. She is indebted to the kindness of some of her companions for many of the anecdotes, as well as for the letters from soldiers who had been under their care; and it is believed that none of the incidents have been overcoloured, as it has been the writer's wish to "nothing extenuate, or aught set down in malice."

March 30th, 1856.

Chapter 1

News of the Battle of the Alma

There are few who will not remember the intense excitement which was roused in England when the newspapers of October 1st announced the Battle of Alma many anxious hopes and fears had been with the army since it left England in March. But months had passed away, little had been done, and expectation had almost ceased when, like the blast of a trumpet, the news of battle and victory rang through the land.

The first burst of exultation had hardly passed away when the lists of killed and wounded arrived, and then the realities of war were brought to almost every English home. The "Gazette" office in London was crowded with inquirers pale with anxiety, who grasped the printed list with trembling hands, and it needed no words to tell the tale revealed to each by the absence or presence of the well-known name in the fatal column.

The *Telegraph* office was crowded by friends anxious to convey glad tidings to country homes. All who had letters hastened to communicate their contents to those who had none. The common bond of sympathy spread through the land; England was like one great family. The lists were followed by the harrowing details of the battlefield, the embarkation of the wounded, and their arrival at the imperfectly prepared hospital at Scutari.

These are too well known to need repetition here; the newspapers were filled with complaints, and their statements produced the same effect everywhere. The first cry was that the wounded had arrived and there was no lint or linen to dress their wounds with. The papers were instantly filled with letters offering both—from house to house, parish to parish, lint was collected in bales and tons till the public were assured on official authority that a further supply was not needed.

But the lint letters were succeeded by others, stating a grave deficiency. Nurses were needed the medical men were overtaxed; the orderlies were ill-accustomed to attend in sickness. Why were the English soldiers to be deprived of the comforts enjoyed by the French?

On the first appearance of sickness at Varna they had sent for Sisters of Charity, and the summons was instantly obeyed, and in bands of twenty-five they went as they were wanted. Why, it was said, are there no such nurses in England? Surely there are women in England as well as in France who would go forth and minister to the wants of the sick and wounded soldiers!

And English women were not wanting. Many was the band that was that week organised for the work; many were the individuals who in their secluded homes determined to offer their services for this purpose, and applied for information and permission to the official authorities.

Amongst other volunteers was the widowed daughter of an Irish nobleman, Lady M—— F——. She engaged three nurses, furnished money for their outfit and expenses, and on the 11th of October she went to Miss Nightingale, then in Harley Street, and requested her to take them out to the East, or to recommend someone else, failing which she was ready to go herself! Subject to the approval of her parents—which was given—Miss Nightingale consented to go, and every preparation was made for her departure on the 17th. Her letter to Mr. Sidney Herbert—asking for government protection—was crossed by one from him, earnestly requesting her to undertake the cause and select her own band.

The scheme from this moment became a public one, and though every day's delay was to be deprecated, it was thought desirable to attempt to procure a larger staff of nurses, and therefore Miss Nightingale's departure was delayed for some days. She appointed two ladies to assist her in the selection of nurses, and while they dealt with individuals she dealt with institutions and communities. From the beginning it was determined that all party feeling was to be merged in the one common bond of alleviating suffering, and in the selection of nurses few questions were asked, and no objections made on the ground of differences of creed or shades of opinion.

The only point on which any stress was laid—and it was laid equally on all—was that proselytising was strictly forbidden.

The Master of St. John's House, Westminster, applied to the Bishop of London, on the 13th, saying he was ready to go out and take seven nurses. The Catholic Bishop of Southwark made a similar application to the War-office on the same day, having completed arrangements for five Sisters of Mercy to start immediately, which they did, but were stopped in Paris, and desired to wait for the whole band, which was then organising under Miss Nightingale. All were to be subject to her in matters relating to the hospital.

With the approval of the Catholic Bishop of Southwark, rules were issued to the Sisters of Mercy for this special service, the first of which was that the Sisters should attend to the corporeal wants of the soldiers, but that they should never introduce religious subjects except with patients of their own faith. The Master of St. John's House accepted Miss Nightingale's terms, after two days consideration.

The institution founded by Mrs. Fry was the first to which Miss Nightingale applied, laying before the Lady Superintendent the terms offered by government; *i.e.*, their not being for the time in connection with any other institution. She replied that none of the nurses would consent to go under such conditions, and the proposal therefore at once fell to the ground. Miss Sellon applied towards the middle of this week, and Miss Nightingale consented to take out eight of her Sisters.

Between sixty and seventy nurses applied to go out—owing to the active kindness of friends who searched London for the purpose. Out of this number eleven were selected with great difficulty, owing to the very low calibre of the applicants. By Saturday, October 21st, the band was completed as follows: Ten Catholic Sisters of Mercy; eight of Miss Sellon's Sisters; six nurses from St. John's; three selected by Lady M. F———; eleven selected from applicants: total, 38. The only additions were Mr. and Mrs. Bracebridge, who most kindly, at the last moment, offered to go and assist Miss Nightingale.

It was on Monday, October 24th, 1854, that this expedition left England, under the escort of Mr. and Mrs. Bracebridge. At Boulogne they were met on landing by the fish-women, who, hearing their mission, insisted on carrying their luggage, gratis, to the Hotel des Bains, where the landlord provided a sumptuous luncheon for the whole party, for which neither he nor anyone in his establishment would accept any remuneration; and he repeated his liberality on the succeeding occasions when bands of nurses passed through on their way to the East.

They proceeded to Marseilles, where the *Vectis* awaited them, and conveyed them, after a stormy passage, to Constantinople, which they reached Saturday, November 4th, and were at once allotted the quarters in the barrack hospital at Scutari which have been thus occupied ever since, (as at 1856).

Meantime the selection of nurses for future bands was left in the hands of Mrs. Sidney Herbert, Miss Stanley, and Miss Jones, Superintendent of St. John's House, Westminster. Each post, each hour, brought fresh applicants; and, as a test of the qualifications of the applicants, it was agreed that, with few exceptions, all should go through training at some of the London Hospitals, and, to facilitate this, St. John's House and St. Saviour's Home, Osnaburgh Street, were opened to receive probationers, and latterly a third institution was established for the same purpose, under the patronage of the Earl of Shaftesbury, in Charlotte Street, Fitzroy Square.

Tidings from the East were eagerly looked for. At last, they came. The nurses had arrived and been well received; and letters were seen from soldiers, from medical men, from military men, all speaking in grateful terms of what women's care already was and would be to them. Many comforts were said to be wanting, and English hearts and English purses were opened to remedy the deficiencies.

The Battles of Balaclava and Inkermann sent down hundreds of sufferers. The medical men in England said the numbers of nurses already gone were but as a drop in the ocean amidst the thousands now in the Eastern hospitals; a second band was to be in readiness to go if sent for. The summons came in a letter from Mr. Bracebridge to Mr. Herbert, who, anxious that as many as possible should benefit by the care of nurses, determined to send out as large a staff as were ready. With as much care as was possible, a selection was made from the registered candidates.

Nine ladies and twenty-two paid nurses were chosen; fifteen Catholic Sisters of Mercy, collected from various convents, under the charge of the superioress of the Convent of Kinsale, placed themselves at the service of the Government, and thus the party was composed. Miss Stanley was requested to go out in charge of them, and place them under Miss Nightingale's care, after which it was her intention to return home. The Honourable Mr. Percy and Dr. Meyer were to accompany them to make arrangements.

On December 1st the party of nurses and ladies assembled at Mr. Sidney Herbert's house in Belgrave Square, and the scene which presented itself was extraordinary; the rooms on the ground floor were turned into a fair, and that not a fancy one—boxes of all sizes, goloshes, cloaks, bonnets, jackets, gowns, collars, caps, lay in admired confusion in all directions. In one room one group were choosing their dresses, and of course short people got long ones, and *vice versa*.

I had better here describe our "Costume." It consisted of a loose wrapping gown of dark grey tweed, a worsted jacket, plain linen collar, and thick white cap; passing over the right shoulder was a broad strip of brown Holland, embroidered in red worsted with the words "Scutari Hospital." A short grey worsted cloak, brown straw bonnet, and veil, completed the dress.

The party were now summoned to stand in a circle to be addressed by Mr. Sidney Herbert. He told us how useful Miss Nightingale and her party were then making themselves in the hospital; he warned us to expect many hardships and discomforts, and to be prepared to witness many scenes of horror; he impressed upon us the necessity of strict obedience to our superiors, and begged us to remember that we all went out on the same footing as hospital nurses, and that no one was to consider herself as in any way above her companions.

We were now summoned by Mrs. Sidney Herbert to sign our agreement, of which the following is a copy:—

> Memorandum of agreement made this 1st day of December 1854, between Miss Nightingale, under the principal medical-officer at ——, on the one part, and —— of —— on the other part. Female nurses being required for the sick and wounded of the British Army serving in the East, the Secretary-at-War has agreed to employ the said —— in the capacity of nurse at a weekly salary of ——, and also to provide board and lodging; also to pay all expenses attendant upon the journeying to or from the present or any future hospital that may be appointed for the accommodation of the sick and wounded of the said army; and to pay all expenses of return to this country, should sickness render it necessary for the said —— to return, save and except such return shall be rendered necessary by the discharge of the said —— for neglect of duty, immoral conduct, or intoxication, in which case the said —— shall forfeit all claim upon the said Miss Nightingale from the period of such discharge. And the said —— hereby agrees to devote her whole time and attention to the purposes aforesaid, under the directions and to the satisfaction of the said Miss Nightingale, the whole of whose orders she undertakes to obey, until discharged by the said Miss Nightingale. Witness ——, December 1st, 1854.

In the case of volunteers, the sentence respecting payment in the agreement was erased.

The last evening was come. Few of those concerned in the morrow's departure slept that night. Last things were to be packed, last words spoken, and ere these were finished it was time to prepare for departure.

Chapter 2

Passage down the Rhone to Valence

Long before dawn on that dark December morning, cabs might have been seen in the silent empty streets, all converging to one point, the London Bridge Station. In the large waiting room at the station the singular party assembled all in costume, and attended by innumerable friends, and when the long train of fifteen nuns, in their black serge dresses, white coifs, and long black veils, joined the party, we formed a group such as was never before seen in London Bridge Station.

Mrs. Sidney Herbert, with thoughtful kindness, brought last gifts and encouraging words to cheer all on their way. Gentlemen perambulated the room with *Illustrated News*, *Punches*, and table-spoons, which latter article seemed to be the last thought for our comfort. We had been informed that whatever luggage we required besides our one box each (which we were never to open from London to Constantinople) we must carry in our hands, consequently we were literally sinking beneath the weight of cloaks, shawls, railway wrappers, baskets, and carpet bags, so that when the cry, "Nurses for Scutari, move on," came, it was with difficulty that many obeyed the summons.

We started about six, heartily cheered by the kind friends who had come to bid us goodbye. We reached Folkestone in two hours, and went straight on board the steamer for Boulogne. It was a lovely morning for the time of year, and Old England's white cliffs stood out brightly in the morning light to receive our looks of farewell. We had a quick but very rough passage, which, with its attendant miseries, there is no need to describe. At Boulogne, we were received by the fish-women, who insisted upon carrying, our luggage from the boat to the station.

An excellent luncheon was kindly provided for us at the *Hotel des Bains*, after which we immediately left for Paris, which we reached late at night. Sunday was spent at Paris without incident. Monday, we travelled to Lyons. December the 5th, early in the morning, we went on board the steamer to go down the Rhone to Valence. A dense fog came on almost immediately after we went on board, in which the steamer ran aground, and delayed us two hours.

When we were once more on our way the fog cleared, and the day proved lovely; we greatly enjoyed our voyage down the many windings of the beautiful river. The Alps in the distance were clearly to be seen. We reached Valence in the afternoon; found, as we expected, that our morning delay had caused us to lose the express train to Marseilles, resolved to proceed by the next train to Avignon, and telegraphed to the hotel there that fifty beds should be prepared. We heard afterwards that the hotel-keeper looked upon it as a hoax; however, he discovered his mistake when the fifty actually arrived.

The hotel was a very old-fashioned one, and the windows of our room looked into a dark and narrow street, so narrow that the houses almost seemed to meet. It was a *fête*-day, and the peasants were dancing by torchlight, and beautiful was the effect of the dark shadows of the houses, and the brilliant glare of light falling on the picturesque dresses of the peasants of Provence.

As we had only to proceed next day to Marseilles, some of our party by rising early managed to visit the Cathedral. It is handsome, but very small in comparison of many in England. It stands in a fine situation, and we were told commands a beautiful view. The pouring rain hid this from our eyes. We arrived at Marseilles at noon, and proceeded to the *Hotel d'Europe*. There was much to be done at Marseilles by those escorting the party; bed and bedding had to be bought and packed, and taken on board ship. The arrangements for the journey through France were made with the utmost liberality, and were carried out with the greatest consideration for the comfort of the party.

At Marseilles the English consul and chaplain were prompt in their offers to render any assistance in their power, and all through France the officials had been most courteous and attentive. We went out shopping for "last thoughts" in spite of the rain, and visited the flower market, which looked as lovely as if it had been summer.

The astonishment of the paid nurses at the *tables d'hôte* used to be our amusement through France. Their views on the subject of French cookery and French customs were not very favourable. "I don't see the use of just eating one thing by itself, and then eating another by itself," says one; "now I likes two or three of them together."

"Yes," we replied, "but that is not the custom in France."

"Well, I means to manage it somehow," says another; "I am a-going to keep this ere fowl on my plate till I get some of that cauliflower," and so she did, in spite of the astonished look of the *garçons*, who had, however, made up their minds that they were a set of wild animals, from whom anything might have been expected.

It was in the afternoon of December the 7th that the party embarked in the *Egyptus*, one of the French mail steamers. She was carrying between two and three hundred French soldiers and officers to the seat of war, and was consequently very much crowded. The nurses expressed great dissatisfaction when they first saw their accommodation in the fore-cabin. The Sisters of Mercy were offered a share of first-class berths, but declined them, preferring to be all together in two of the fore-cabins. The ladies were all in saloon cabins.

The very first night was stormy, and it appeared the *Egyptus* was out of repair; and but for the great demand for troop ships she would have been in the docks six months before. Her decks required caulking, and nothing was secure. Press of weather drove the *Egyptus* into Hyeres for some hours.

Towards evening of the 8th, the gale went down, and we proceeded on our way. The French soldiers all slept on deck, and they used to go to sleep at dusk; so, after dinner, the favourite time on board ship for taking a walk, one could not pace five yards without stumbling upon a Frenchman wrapped in his grey coat: he never seemed to mind it or even to wake. A miserable-looking set of boys were those poor French soldiers.

We had rather rough weather until the night of December 11th, when the sea became quite calm, and not long after midnight the announcement was made that we were passing Stromboli. Many of us went on deck. We passed close by the island, which is like a rock glowing with fire in the midst of the ocean. Every now and then a bright flame burst out, blazed for a moment, and then disappeared; and then the rock glowed again so intensely as if it would almost burn and consume itself; and yet there it has burnt from age to age, and will still burn on.

At daylight we anchored off Messina; and after some delay, before we found out there was no quarantine, most of us went on shore. The Sisters of Mercy remained on board—they considered it contrary to their rule to leave the vessel except on business.

Great was the enjoyment of that day. Winter seemed to have vanished. It was like the loveliest summer's day, so bright, and fresh, and sweet. Groves loaded with oranges and lemons, the bright blue Mediterranean calm as a lake, the mountains of Calabria in the distance, and the picturesque town of Messina itself—all this lay spread before us as we stood on the steps of the church of San Angelo.

We went into the church, and there the beauty of art tried hard to rival that of nature. The church is very small; but the interior is entirely of mosaic, in excellent preservation; the roof fresco. It was a spot in which one could have spent hours in delight and wonder at its marvellous beauty; but our time of course was short. We went further up the hill, to the Capuchin monastery, into the garden of which the gentlemen of our party were admitted, and they brought from it handsful of oranges, given by the good monks to comfort the ladies for not being permitted to enter. We saw their chapel, however, which was poor and small.

Descending the hill into the town, we visited the Cathedral. Over the west door is a most beautiful piece of sculpture. Over the high altar is a small picture of the Madonna and Child, believed to have been painted by St. Luke, and accordingly preserved in a silver case, set with precious stones; so carefully preserved is it that we could hardly see the picture.

The archbishop's throne was hung with Tyrian purple, what we should call a very pale lilac. Leaving the cathedral, we walked through the streets to regain the shore. They were filthy beyond description. It is said to be the dirtiest continental town; but even the dirt does not take off the picturesque effect. The very tall white houses, with draperies of the brightest colours hanging out of the windows; the shops, also hanging out their goods of various hues; the costume of the people, and the glimpses as we turned down every *strada* of the lovely bay, made our walk through Messina a delightful one.

Towards evening we went on board, and soon after sailed. A second storm occurred after leaving Messina, and a terrible night and day followed. For those who never moved from their berths, in the saloon cabins it did not much signify, but the unhappy occupants of fore-cabins were far worse off. In the middle of the night the skylight was torn off, and the sea poured into the cabins occupied by the nuns and nurses. The nurses on this occasion behaved extremely well, no murmurs escaped their lips. Gratefully they received every attempt to better their condition; and the ensuing night, of their own accord, they offered up a thanksgiving to Almighty God for their safe deliverance from the perils of the storm.

The scene of the storm was past description, the men darted in to bale out the water, some were too sick to care for anything, some called "*garçon*" and others began to prepare for instant death. When daylight came the poor Sisters found that the sea had penetrated into their trunks; and books and clothes, and ornaments for their chapel, were entirely spoiled. The misery the poor Sisters endured, and most patiently, during this voyage was untold. No breakfast could be got that day; so sick and well fasted till dinner time, when the storm began to abate, and the night of December the 11th was spent in the harbour of Navarino.

On December the 15th we anchored off the Piraeus; great delay was caused by our getting on shore, owing to quarantine having been established for cholera some time back. It did not, however, then exist, so we landed at last, with peremptory orders from the captain to be on board again by noon.

Upon landing, we found it would be out of the question to visit Athens, which is a distance of six miles from the Piraeus. We contented ourselves with driving about the green hills and gazing on the distant view. We returned on board at noon; but the despatches for which the captain was obliged to wait did not come till 4 p.m., so that we might have gone to Athens after all. We had good weather after leaving the Piraeus; Saturday, December the 16th, we passed the plains of Troy, one evening at sunset (they were covered with indescribably lovely tints of soft lilac: that is the only expression which seems to describe it, but it was a colour rarely if ever seen before), and entered the Dardanelles.

It was dark before we reached Gallipoli, where we anchored for some hours. Two French *Soeurs de la Charité* came on board to proceed to Constantinople. Many of us had never seen *les Soeurs de la Charité* before; we found on inquiry that they belonged to the order of St. Vincent de Paul, and are bound only by annual vows. The order was founded two hundred years ago, and they wear the peasant dress of that period, consisting of grey serge, with jacket and loose sleeves, and a large stiff white peasant cap, of which it is said one of the kings of France invented the shape by folding his dinner napkin into it.

The ship was so crowded that there was not a single berth for the *soeurs*, and they were quite contented to sit up all night, but they received a warm welcome from the Sisters of Mercy, who invited them to share their small cabin for the night. Next morning some of our party who could converse in French were anxious to talk to them, but they were prevented. The French officers and soldiers on board evidently looked upon *les soeurs* as their exclusive property, and treated them with affectionate respect; immediately they made their appearance on deck they were surrounded by their countrymen, who did not relinquish them until we arrived at our destination. The last day of voyage had arrived; Sunday the 17th found the *Egyptus* rolling through the Sea of Marmora.

About noon the first haze of Constantinople appeared on the horizon, and every eye was fixed in that direction. The first distant view disappointed us. But it is only on rounding Seraglio Point, and entering the Golden Horn, that, as the eye slowly gathers in the wonderful extent of mosques and minarets, the varied shipping, the palaces and the groves of cypresses, the marvellous beauty of the imperial city bursts forth. No travellers had before, we supposed, so quickly called off their attention from the beautiful panorama of Constantinople, to gaze on objects which, though possessing no beauty, were full of interest to them—the hospitals of Scutari, the goal of their long travel, and our future home.

Both stand in commanding positions near the edge of the cliff overhanging the Sea of Marmora, looking upon the Golden Horn, Seraglio Point, and the city in the distance; how our hearts burned and yearned to be in those hospitals, to be accomplishing the object for which we had left our dear country and our loved homes, to be soothing in some small degree a portion of the mighty mass of suffering collected in those wards. Such were our thoughts as we slowly passed Scutari and anchored in the Golden Horn.

The vast collection of shipping which fills the bay adds greatly to the extraordinary beauty of the scene. At this time the flags of all nations except the Russian were flying. The fairy-like *caiques* shot rapidly by (even the commonest of these boats were richly ornamented with, carving); then came the *pasha's caiques* with their bright cushions and carpets, their six rowers all dressed in white with the crimson *fez*, the *pasha* himself sitting in state with his pipe-bearer behind him; then came the heavy passage boats loaded with passengers and luggage, among the former, numbers of Turkish women closely wrapped in their *feridgee* and *yachmae*; the rowers of these passage boats rise from them seats each time they raise their oar, so that their progress is slow and tedious. These were some of the strange sights we watched that Sunday afternoon from the deck of the *Egyptus*.

One of the gentlemen of our escort went in a *caique* to Scutari to announce our arrival to Miss Nightingale. All agreed it was necessary we should sleep on board that night. The passengers who were not of our party soon went on shore, while we sat watching the sunset as its golden light fell upon tower and minaret, and shed a sort of halo over the queenly city. We watched till the stars came out; then the moon rose, and beautiful indeed looked Constantinople bathed in its soft silver rays.

Mr. Bracebridge came on board that evening and brought news that the next morning the admiral's small steamer would be alongside to convey us, not to Scutari, but to a house belonging to the ambassador at Therapia—a village fifteen miles up the Bosphorus, on the European side—the reason of this change being that there was no room for us at present at Scutari.

This news insensibly cast a damp over our spirits, although it seemed but reasonable that we should be delayed for a few days. The French Sisters of Charity, who have a large convent in Galata, sent to offer to receive the Sisters of Mercy for a short time, for, it being the Christmas holidays, and their boarding-school having broken up, they were enabled to spare them a room in their generally well-crowded convent.

As we all looked forward to a week's delay as the longest possible time, this offer was accepted, and next morning the party separated. The nuns proceeded to Galata, the ladies and nurses, under Miss Stanley's charge, to Therapia, the gentlemen to an hotel in Pera. On December the 18th, with thankful hearts for our merciful preservation through a perilous voyage, we quitted the *Egyptus*, and the little steamer quickly conveyed us to Therapia.

It was a pleasant passage; the banks of the Bosphorus are thickly crowded with houses, which often overhang the waters. Here and there a small Turkish cemetery, with its dark cypresses and gaily-coloured tombstones, or a *Sultan's* palace, with its terraced gardens, or mosques and minarets of snowy whiteness, diversify the scene; on the high points of the hills, are the picturesque kiosks, or summer houses, the many windings of the Bosphorus, the dark hills and valleys between, the varied colouring of the wooden houses on either side, made our passage up to Therapia seem like a series of pictures.

CHAPTER 3

Continued Delay at Therapia

We reached Therapia about eleven in the morning, and the steamer anchored at the quay immediately before the house we were to occupy, which was the summer residence of the *attachés* of the British Embassy. The quay, which divides the house from the Bosphorus, is about four yards wide. Entering the garden and ascending a long flight of steps led us into a long hall, from which various rooms opened.

All the rooms in the house were on this floor; the kitchen, as in most Turkish houses, separate from the house. The house was only partially furnished, but all deficiencies were supplied that afternoon from Constantinople, and the evening was spent in arrangements.

Miss Stanley refused assistance from the English hotel in Therapia, thinking it best to employ the paid nurses in the household work which was to be performed. But now the evils of the equality system began to appear. The ladies had suffered by it through the journey, for having no authority to restrain the hired nurses they were compelled to listen to the worst language, and to be treated not unfrequently with coarse insolence. Whispers were heard amongst them that first evening, that they had come out to nurse the soldiers and not to sweep, wash, and cook.

The following morning, after breakfast, Miss Stanley assembled the whole party, and after returning thanks for the termination of the long and stormy voyage, she addressed the nurses, informing them that she could not tell how long we might be delayed at Therapia, but whether for a long or short time she trusted we should live together in peace and harmony, "serving one another by love," each assisting to the best of her power in the work of the house as she should allot to them. She reminded them of the serious and important work they had come out to perform, and how much depended on their own conduct. She then assigned to each their work.

The discontent was not altogether quelled by this kind address; most of the paid nurses performed their work with an air of infinite condescension. One was asked what she could do in helping the work of the house. Could she wash? No! Iron? No! Then what could she do? "Make a poultice!" she replied. But as there were none to make, Mrs. —— retired to her room, and employed herself about her own devices as long as we stayed at Therapia. Some few of the nurses worked hard and willingly for the public good.

Therapia is the summer residence of the English and French ministers; a good many country houses and a large hotel complete the fashionable part. All these are built on the quay. The British embassy stands a little further back, with a beautiful terraced garden, ascending from whence one reaches a high point, on which is planted the flag staff. From here there is a magnificent view. One can see the entrance to the Black Sea; the village of Buyukdere, round the point; the many windings of the stream; the dark hills on the Asiatic side, and the Giant's Hill just opposite, the highest point of this part of the country.

Hills rise so immediately round Therapia in Turkey.

Around the house in which we lived was a large garden, at the extreme end of which, quite hidden among the trees, was a small house, the summer residence of Lord Napier, Secretary to the Embassy; the use of this house also was offered to us by Lord Stratford de Redcliffe, and it was assigned by Miss Stanley for the use of the nuns, after they had been a few days at Galata. After passing the *Hotel d'Angleterre* the stone quay ends, and the village begins, which consists of a few wretched shops, some *cafés*, a French *magasin*, and a small Greek church.

After passing through the village the quay recommences, there are a few better sort of houses, then two large buildings, which were at that time converted into British and French naval hospitals, and the *Sultan's* palace: eventually this last became the British naval convalescent hospital, but at the time we were at Therapia they possessed only the one building.

On Christmas-day there was no English service. The chaplain being indisposed, prayers were read at home, and we adorned the rooms with green, sang carols, and tried to make ourselves believe it was really Christmas-day. Lady Stratford, with her well-known kindness, sent up mince pies and plum-pudding, with kind Christmas wishes. We were very grateful for her kind remembrance of us, but our Christmas was a dreary one. The joyous sounds of English Christmases were ringing in our ears, and it was an oppressive thought to remember that through the length and breadth of that fair land, save from the few bodies of strangers who dwelt in it for a time, there went up no sounds of rejoicing for the glad tidings of great joy. No bells rang out to welcome the birthday of the King of kings. (The Greek Church celebrates Christmas twelve days later.)

Therapia is quite a Greek village. The services at the Greek church are most curious and picturesque. The church itself is small and common-looking outside, inside much decorated with pictures, chandeliers, great candlesticks, and painted pillars, all rather tawdry when looked into except the rood screen, which is one of the most beautiful pieces of carving I ever beheld; it reaches entirely to the ceiling, and it is only in the space above the door which admits the priest into the chancel that you catch a view of the altar.

This space is generally covered with an embroidered curtain only withdrawn at mass. The service was most extraordinary. Two priests stood in stalls in the nave with large books, out of which they chanted (at least I suppose it was intended for such), but it sounded like the most dismal howling. It was an indescribably discordant noise. The congregation employed themselves in walking up to two or three little pictures and kissing them repeatedly. They then crossed themselves a great many times, and lighted the smallest wax tapers in the world, which they stuck by the side of the same little pictures.

Then the curtain before the altar was drawn back, and the priest appeared in an under robe of dark brown and fur, and an outer one of crimson and gold. He was an old man, with a long white beard. He brought with him a censer, with which he incensed the people, then the host was carried round the church, the people forming into two lines as it passed, the men bowing the head, the women bending down till their hands touched the ground—they never kneel. We could not understand the service; it did not seem like the celebration of mass. The priest at the altar was saying prayers, but the two in the nave would not let his voice be heard: they continued their musical sounds so as to drown all others.

It was certainly a most striking scene. The Greek men are a handsome race, very different to the women, who are extremely plain; even the commonest race of men are all like pictures—the dress doubtless has something to do with it. On Sundays and *fête*-days it is so picturesque; the full trousers gathered in at the knee, the tunic of the same colour', perhaps of deep blue, showing the embroidered vest, the bright-coloured scarf round the waist, and the crimson *fez*. Nothing can equal getting through the streets of Constantinople at this season. The way of walking is for each to hold by the other's cloak, and to walk in a string; what with the mud and the constant danger of being run over, walking in Constantinople is rather a laborious occupation.

Some of our party took an excursion to the Giant's Hill, on the Asiatic shore. It is the highest point of the hills of the Bosphorus, and from its summit there is a fine view of the Black Sea, the Golden Horn, and the Sea of Marmora. When they were all safe at home again, they were told they might have been carried off by the *Bashi Bazouks*, and kept till they were ransomed! Our readers may believe this as they please.

Our life flowed on monotonously enough at Therapia—ironing the clothes which the nurses condescended to wash for us, taking a walk on the quay when weather permitted, and writing home, were the employments day after day. How long the weeks seemed! The constant expectation contributed to heighten this feeling. Every Sunday we hoped the next would see us at work, and Sunday after Sunday brought disappointment.

Miss Stanley answered all our inquiries as to the delay by stating that, in consequence of the arrival of eight hundred sick from the camp, there was no room for us at Scutari, and we were to remain where we were till arrangements were made for our employment.

The occasional amusement to some of us was shopping. We not understanding a word of Greek, and the shopkeepers knowing no English, the bargain was conducted entirely by signs; for instance, the supply of flat irons being very insufficient, one of the party volunteered to buy one; everyone said she would never find it. She resolved to try, so she pointed to article after article to try and represent what she wanted, but in vain.

At last, she laid one end of her cloak on the counter and ironed it with her hand. The Greek clapped his hands, while his eyes sparkled, and away he rushed into some back region and brought out the oldest, rustiest affair in the shape of an iron ever beheld—a treasure to us, however; he asked thirty-four *piastres* (9*s*.), and took eighteen *piastres* (3*s*.), of course a great deal too much for it.

Then we discovered an old tin-man; he was a Turk by the bye (and he lived in a barrel), and he made vessels in tin, which articles it was advisable after buying not to place too near the fire, as their construction was not very strong. The old Turk made treasures for us in the shape of tin pots or jugs, which would hold about a pint; in these we could heat hot water.

The Protestant afternoon service on Sunday (there were no morning prayers) was in one of the wards of the naval hospital. We suppose no other place could have been found; but it was a trial to go there— the smell and atmosphere were both so unhealthy. This condition of the atmosphere of these hospitals arose from the number of cases of frost-bites then under treatment. The arrangements for ventilation were good, and every possible care and attention was shown to the patients.

The Catholic services were performed in a ward of the French naval hospital, the atmosphere of which was even worse than the British. Every morning the long train of the fifteen Sisters of Mercy was seen slowly wending their way thither; they never, except for this purpose, went beyond the grounds of the embassy.

Our services as nurses were offered to the authorities at the British naval hospital, but were declined, in consequence of their then expecting a party of their own, sent out, of course, by the Admiralty. In the meantime, the surgeons said that if any of the nurses could wash for their hospital, they would be very thankful, as their washing was three months in arrear. It is a matter of great difficulty to get washing done in Turkey. The surgeons had hired two Maltese women to wash, but both soon ran away.

Miss Stanley appointed some nurses for this work, and a volunteer wished to join; she said as she could not nurse soldiers she would wash for sailors, and for about a month from morning to night she fulfilled her task, which was not a light one. There would be few ladies whose health would have enabled them to undertake such a labour. Two or three of the ladies daily visited the naval hospital to talk to the men, and write letters for them.

They also sent large baskets full of the patients' linen to our house to be mended, and in the evenings, we sat round the table in the hall at our work, while one of the party read aloud. Sometimes such a treasure as an English newspaper fell into our hands. It was astonishing how precious a scrap of home news became. We were quite sorry when the mending was done, but with so many hands it did not take long.

Our spirits were beginning to rise at the prospect of work, for negotiations were opened for nurses to be sent to Balaclava; and we heard it was intended to remove the Russian prisoners from the barracks at Koulali, and occupy that building as a British hospital. There was a good deal of sickness among us, not of a serious character, but climatising. The naval surgeons attended those who were ill, and never can they forget the friendly kindness and attention which they received from these gentlemen. In them we indeed found friends in a foreign land.

The weather continued very variable; sometimes the cold was intense; snow would lie on the ground for several days. We suffered much from cold, not that it was so intense as some of the severe frosts in England, but the want of means to warm oneself added so greatly to it. In our large house were two stoves only, which gave but little heat. In the house occupied by the Sisters of Mercy there were no stoves, nothing but charcoal brasiers. It should be remembered that these houses are built solely for summer residences, and are never inhabited in the winter. Blankets we did not possess, so railway wrappers and cloaks were useful beyond expression. One stove was supposed to warm the long hall, which it certainly did not do.

One night someone sitting beside the stove in the hall saw smoke issuing from under the stove plate; she gave the alarm, and we discovered that the plate was laid upon the floor, the woodhouse being underneath. In half-an-hour more the whole would have been in flames, and we turned out on a bitter cold winter evening. As all the houses were built of wood, and there were no engines, the destruction would have been great. Fortunately, we were in time to stop it, the only bad consequence being that we were forbidden to have any fire in it at all till the plate was raised on stones from the flooring. This simple operation taking a long time in Turkey, we were for several days in the coldest weather without any fire save a charcoal brasier.

Sometimes after a severe frost would come a day of spring more bright and lovely than any in England. One Sunday was like this; we watched the fishing from the window. A number of *caiques* all darted to one particular spot just before our windows, where a shoal of fishes happened to be at little distances; a *caique* or two were scattered here and there, but the group in the midst was the most remarkable: they struggled and fought who should throw in their nets. It seemed as if they would overturn the *caiques*.

At last, in went net after net, and up they came brimful of little silver fishes, and they emptied their nets into the bottom of the boat, and plunged them in again. The heap of fishes glistening in the sunshine, the bright blue Bosphorus smooth as a lake, the dark hills in the distance, the curiously shaped boats and the picturesque dress of the boatmen, their shrill voices, rapid actions, and foreign language, made a picture not easily forgotten, and brought to mind the celebrated cartoon of the miraculous draught. We pleased ourselves with comparing the scene before us to that of the blue lake of Galilee, the eastern hills and Hebrew fishermen.

Immediately behind the Barrack Hospital, quite at the foot of the hills, almost secluded from sight, is the British naval burying ground. It looked a dreary spot then; the grass had not grown over the graves, the rain had made the clay mould wet and muddy. No stone marked who rested there—no sign that they whose remains slept there lay down in a better hope than the poor Turks who were buried close by; no sign that the sleepers were enshrined in the hearts of their country and died in her service.

About halfway up the hill was the French naval burying ground, almost every grave marked by its little wooden cross, with the name of him who was buried there, the ship he belonged to, and the date of his death, written on it. True, the wood would in time sink into the earth, but it was pleasing to see the care and thought bestowed. We did not like the contrast between the countries, and the ladies of our party determined to raise a monument to the memories of the sailors and marines who were buried in our burial ground.

We had to ask permission for this from the Admiralty, and therefore we could not see our wish carried out before we left Therapia. It was our unanimous wish that it should be a cross to distinguish the burial ground as a Christian one. It now stands in Therapia's British naval burying ground. We afterwards heard that it was badly constructed, and badly placed by the sculptor; nevertheless, we trusted the friends of those whose bodies rest beneath that foreign sod would not despise our offering. The stone is inscribed with these words:—

> This stone is raised to the memory of the sailors and marines buried in this graveyard (their names are then inscribed in order) by their countrywomen.

On the arms of the cross are engraven the words:

> "I am the Resurrection and the Life."

Miss Stanley was frequently absent from us for a day or two at a time; her anxiety to have us released from our very unpleasant position was very great. She went frequently to the British embassy at Pera, and met there with much kindness from Lady Stratford, who interested herself warmly in procuring employment for our band. Miss Stanley also went often to Scutari, to try and make arrangements for the reception of some more of her nurses.

During Miss Stanley's absences our anxiety to know our fate grew very intense, and we used to watch for the steamer by which we expected her return eagerly. Two steamers went daily from Buyukdere to Pera, touching at Therapia; one returned at four in the afternoon, the other half-an-hour later. When it touched the quay, loaded with passengers, we looked anxiously for Miss Stanley, or Nicola, the interpreter, who would perhaps bring us letters if she were not there. If she were there she was instantly surrounded by the number of expectant ladies. "Oh, Miss Stanley, what news? Are we going away? Are we to be sent home? What can it all mean?"

Miss Stanley's unvarying answer was that we must be patient, that obstacles were in our way which must be removed ere we could gain admittance to the hospital; she would never say in what these obstacles consisted, and very patiently withstood all our questioning. She was deservedly much beloved by all for her just government of the community, her uniform sweetness of temper and thoughtful kindness for all—but many and bitter were the complaints made of her "vagueness." We could not find out from her why we were detained, and whose fault it was, and that vexed us sadly.

Great excitement also was roused amongst us when the summons came for one or two of the party to leave us for Scutari. This happened twice. Two nurses who were known as very good surgical nurses were sent for. One of these women happened to be a soldier's wife; her chief motive for coming out was to be near her husband. Her friends at home tried to dissuade her from coming, pointing out how very unlikely it was that she should be able to meet with him. She persisted in her wish, and curiously enough the day we entered the Golden Horn he among other sick came down from the camp to Scutari.

She did not know this for a week after, and was then prevented by her own illness from going to him for another week. She went at length, and found him dying. She waited on him the last two days of his life, and then after his death remained as nurse for some months.

Next, one of the ladies of our party was sent for, Miss Nightingale wishing her to take the office of superintendent of the nurses in the General Hospital, Scutari. Great was our anxiety to know what became of our companions. As soon as they left us, we heard no more of them; they wrote short notes, saying nothing of what we most wanted to know, *viz.*, their work.

Next came a great move; two ladies, five nuns, and several paid nurses were sent for. We were told at the time that this hand composed the whole of those who would be admitted into Scutari Hospital, the rest of the party were to be divided between Balaclava and Koulali, and we waited with as much patience as we could for the conclusion of the arrangements which would open these new fields of labour to us.

Miss Stanley was requested to take the office of superintendent of nurses at Koulali; and she consented to delay her return home for a time and to start the nursing there.

About Balaclava there were many and various opinions; many thought that the Crimea was not sufficiently in the hands of the allies to make it safe for women to go there, that in the event of an attack they would only be a burden, while the hardships they would have to endure would be too great. We were told that, though Miss Nightingale did not forbid it, she would not sanction it. The point was, I believe, decided by Lord Raglan's expressed wish for the assistance of eight nurses.

Miss Nightingale appointed, as superintendent of the Balaclava nursing staff, one of Miss Sellon's Sisters under her charge; her seven companions were to be selected from those of our party who should volunteer to go; there were nine volunteers, seven were selected by Miss Stanley, two ladies, five nurses. Great preparations were made for their departure; *rumour* (our only source of information) said that they would find nothing but unfurnished huts at Balaclava; and so, the village was ransacked for cooking utensils, as far as the miserable shops of Therapia would furnish; bedsteads and bedding were packed, and all was ready.

A note from Miss Stanley (who was staying at the embassy in Pera) announced that passages were taken on board the *Melbourne* for the party for Balaclava; that the superintendent would go on board in the Golden Horn; that the *Melbourne* would lie off Therapia sufficient time to allow the party to go on board, but that all the luggage must be embarked in *caiques*, and those lie off the house ready to start as soon as the *Melbourne* should lay to. She was to sail on the 15th of January; early on that day the *caique* with well-loaded luggage lay off the quay before the house.

The party were all ready dressed, and every eye watched the vessels as they passed; but the day wore on, and no ship lay to off Therapia. When night came on a general sense of disappointment fell on all the Balaclava party. We had grown so familiar with suspense and disappointment that they were not satisfied with our assurances that ships hardly ever sailed on the day they professed to do; they could not be persuaded but that some obstacle had arisen. When the next morning came, six of the party declared they could not bear to spend the day as they had done the preceding one, with their bonnets on, watching the ships; they would employ themselves in some way, and be ready at five minutes' notice.

One lady of the party, the one who had washed at the hospital, and who was especially distinguished for her self-devotion, had been from the first most anxious to go to Balaclava; she was sorely afraid some obstacle had arisen from this delay in the *Melbourne*, and she would not wait like the others, but dressed ready as, before.

The day was stormy, the Bosphorus very rough. Nicola came directly after breakfast to say that the *caidjee* declared it was too rough for him to lie off the quay; he must go into a little bay opposite the village. Our friend would not lose sight of her boxes, so she insisted upon going thither with him, and seated herself among the boxes in the *caique*, and patiently kept her place the whole morning. As little groups of our party passed down the quay for walking or shopping, there they found her settled. How we laughed! She did not care a bit, but took it all in good part.

To crown the whole, early in the afternoon a vessel was seen in the distance; it would have taken nearly an hour to ascertain whether it was the *Melbourne*—we could not even see her colours; but our friend could not wait, so off the *caique* and boxes and lady went, over the billows of the Bosphorus, which were many and fierce that day, till it lay alongside the vessel. The lady boarded her and found she was French, the captain very polite, but could give her no information respecting the *Melbourne*.

Again, the lady seated herself in her *caique*; we watching from our windows saw the little dark speck dancing on the waves. "Surely she is coming home now," we said. "She certainly will be drowned on this rough day;" and, exclaimed one of the Balaclava party, "She has got all our boxes with her, and *they* will all be lost!"

Another sail was seen on the horizon, and we saw the little speck turn in that direction, and soon lie alongside this vessel. Though we were really alarmed at the freak, it was impossible to help laughing at the pertinacity with which she pursued her object. At this juncture one of the naval surgeons came in and joined in the laugh, but soon said, "Really it is too rough for such an adventure. I hope she has two *caidjee* with her."

"No, indeed; only one," we answered.

He instantly ran out and ordered a *caique* with two rowers to follow our adventurous friend. However, before it could reach her, she had returned in safety, and her mind at rest. The second vessel was English, and the officer in charge knew the *Melbourne* was still in dock, and had not finished coaling. So now all were satisfied, and it was well, for three more days of suspense were their portion. At length, on the 19th at noon, the *Melbourne* lay off Therapia, and the party were soon safely on board.

CHAPTER 4

The General Hospital, Scutari

The day at last arrived when the establishment at Therapia was finally broken up. Seven had gone to Balaclava; three hired nurses had been sent home (one from ill-health, two from their habits of intoxication); two more hired nurses had been sent to private cases at Pera, while waiting for Government work (they afterwards joined the Koulali nursing staff); eighteen were received at Scutari, and the remaining sixteen under Miss Stanley's charge, went to Koulali. We will now follow the footsteps of those proceeding to Scutari. We landed at the wharf, and climbing the steep hill found ourselves at the main guard or principal entrance to Scutari barrack hospital.

The hospital is an immense square building; three long corridors run completely round it, and it is three storeys high. Numberless apartments open out of all these corridors, which are called wards. At each corner of the building is a tower. The main guard divides A corridor; turning to the left after passing through one or two divisions from which the guard rooms open, we came to the sick.

To avoid the cold air of the long corridor, wooden partitions were put up, and the spaces between these were called divisions. We made our way through the double row of sick to the tower at the corner (Miss Nightingale's quarters); the smell in this corridor of sick was quite overpowering—they were almost all surgical cases, which, I suppose, was partly the cause.

On arriving at Miss Nightingale's quarters, we entered the large kitchen or hall, from which all the other rooms opened. There were four rooms on the lower storey occupied as follows:—Mr. and Mrs. Bracebridge in one; Miss Nightingale in another; the five nuns in the third; fourteen nurses and one lady in the last. A staircase led up the tower to two other rooms; the first occupied by the Sisters from Miss Sellon's and other ladies, the second by the nurses belonging to St. John's Training Institution.

The kitchen was used as Miss Nightingale's extra-diet kitchen. From this room were distributed quantities of arrowroot, sago, rice puddings, jelly, beef-tea, and lemonade, upon requisitions made by the surgeons. This caused great comings to and fro; numbers of orderlies were waiting at the door with requisitions. One of the nuns or a lady received them, and saw they were signed and countersigned, and then served them.

We used, among ourselves, to call this kitchen the tower of Babel, from the variety of languages spoken in it and the confusion. In fact, in the middle of the day everything and everybody seemed to be there. Boxes, parcels, bundles of sheets, shirts, and old linen and flannels; tubs of butter, sugar, bread, kettles, saucepans, heaps of books, and of all kinds of rubbish, besides the "diets," which were being dispensed; then the people, ladies, nuns, nurses, orderlies, Turks, Greeks, French and Italian servants, officers, and others waiting to see Miss Nightingale; all passing to and fro, all intent upon their own business, and all speaking their own language.

The ladies' quarters were the first room upstairs. It was a good-sized one, with eight windows, and having a fine view of the sea. A divan ran round the room, covered with stuffed cushions, which, together with the matting, were well furnished with fleas. A number of rats also lived in the divan and wainscoting, and took nightly promenades about the room.

On Tuesday mornings a Turk came to hoist the Turkish flag from the summit of the tower. He therefore passed through our room at sunrise to put it up, and at sunset to take it down: he always omitted the ceremony of knocking at the door, and as he always took off his shoes also, it was not very easy to discern his approach.

Two days after my arrival, Miss Nightingale sent for me to go with her round the hospital. (Miss Nightingale generally visited her special cases at night). We went round the whole of the second storey, into many of the wards and into one of the upper corridors. It seemed an endless walk, and it was one not easily forgotten. As we slowly passed along, the silence was profound; very seldom did a moan or cry from those multitudes of deeply suffering ones fall on our ears. A dim light burnt here and there. Miss Nightingale carried her lantern, which she would set down before she bent over any of the patients. I much admired Miss Nightingale's manner to the men—it was so tender and kind.

All the corridors were thickly lined with beds laid on low trestles raised a few inches from the ground. In the wards a divan runs round the room, and on this were laid the straw beds, and the sufferers on them. The hospital was crowded to its fullest extent. The building, which has since been reckoned to hold, with comfort, seventeen hundred men, then held between three and four thousand.

Miss Nightingale assigned me my work—it was half A corridor, the whole of B, half C, the whole of I, (on the third storey), and all the wards leading out of these respective corridors; in each corridor there were fifteen of these, except in No. 1, where there were only six. This work I was to share with another lady and one nurse. The number of patients under our charge was, as far as I could reckon, about fifteen hundred.

Miss Nightingale told us only to attend to those in the divisions of those surgeons who wished for our services. She said the staff-surgeon of the division was willing we should work under him, and she charged us never to do anything for the patients without the leave of the doctors.

When we had gone round the hospital, we came out of A corridor upon the main guard.

The blast of cold air from the entrance was refreshing after the overpowering smell of the wards. The corridors of the lower story were under the charge of Miss E——, from Miss Sellon's, assisted by nurses; the remainder of A, under Sister M. S——, of the Bermondsey nuns; the upper corridors, except No. I, under another nun. Several nurses were engaged in different divisions of C corridor; the rest in the diet kitchen.

It seems simply impossible to describe Scutari Hospital at this time. Far abler pens have tried, and all, in some measure, failed; for what an eye-witness saw was past description. Even those who read the harrowing accounts in the *Times* and elsewhere, could not have imagined the full horror of the reality. As we passed the corridors, we asked ourselves if it was not a terrible dream. When we woke in the morning, our hearts sank down at the thought of the woe we must witness that day.

At night we lay down wearied beyond expression; but not so much from physical fatigue, though that was great, as from the sickness of heart from living amidst that mass of hopeless suffering. On all sides prevailed the utmost confusion—whose fault it was I cannot tell—clear heads have tried to discover in vain: probably the blame should have been shared by all the departments of the hospital.

It is necessary here to particularise some of the hospital rules to give an idea of our work. First, the diet roll. In London hospitals a diet card for each patient hangs at the head of his bed, and any alteration in it is generally, if not always, made by the house-surgeon. In military hospitals the diet roll is a book of foolscap paper, with a sheet for each day, and small divisions for each diet. Whatever is inserted in the diet rolls (as in all hospitals), cannot be furnished till the next day.

In military hospitals a man is placed either on full, half, low, or spoon diet. If a man is on full diet, one column is sufficient, as by it is understood that he is to have daily 1lb. of meat, *ditto* of bread, *ditto* of potatoes, and two pints of tea, also half-a-pint of porter. Half-diet is exactly the half of this. Low-diet the half again of that. Spoon-diet is simply one pound of bread and two pints of tea; but it has this difference, that the surgeon may give a man on spoon-diet extras; but for any patient on full, half, or low diet he may not: nor may the surgeons order more than two or three extras to the spoon-diets—the extras at this time were fowls, mutton chops, potatoes, milk, eggs, arrowroot, rice, sago, and lemons for lemonade.

Before the diet roll could be sent into the purveyor's stores it had to be signed by the assistant-surgeon in charge of the patients, whose names were inserted on it, and then it had to be countersigned by the staff-surgeon of the division. The staff-surgeon being the assistant-surgeon's superior officer, and medical etiquette entirely sinking in military discipline, it is quite possible that an assistant-surgeon may be called to account for any extravagance in the diet roll, and this sometimes happened, for extravagance seemed to be the great bugbear of our Eastern hospitals.

The diet rolls were written by the sergeants or corporals appointed as ward masters; if they made any mistake (which they very often did) there was no redress. If they had forgotten to insert an extra to such a name, he must for that day go without it.

The purveying department was at that time in a most inefficient state; constantly the requirements of the diet rolls were not complied with, the stores were given out most irregularly, the orderlies were often obliged to go down to the store-rooms at four a.m. to draw the rations for breakfast; the last of the hand would not be served till past seven a.m. The men's dinners, which ought to have come at twelve, often did not come till five or six p.m.—three p.m. was thought excellent time. Very often we saw the orderlies cutting up the carcases of sheep in the corridor close by the beds in which were men suffering from every form of disease.

Of course, many cases must arise in which the patients are in such a state that their diet must be altered or added to that day. The means of doing this is by a requisition signed by the assistant-surgeon. He must write a separate requisition for each man, and after he has signed it, it is taken to the staff-surgeon to be countersigned, and then to the stores.

This regulation, and indeed all others, were made for military hospitals in an ordinary state, when the buildings only hold the numbers, they are intended for, where every department is sufficiently supplied with people to work it, where extreme cases are to be counted in each ward by ones and twos, and can then of course receive the full attention of the surgeon; but these same laws brought to bear in the Eastern hospitals in that unprecedented time of distress became useless—extreme cases in Scutari were counted by one or two hundreds—it was a matter of impossibility for surgeons to write requisitions enough for their patients' wants, especially as they had to be countersigned by the staff-surgeon, a man having a large charge besides many other duties, and who was never sure of being found in any one place after the regular hours of going his rounds. The purveying department was also so utterly inefficient that constantly requisitions were signed and sent in, and then not honoured.

Miss Nightingale's diet kitchen has been before mentioned; the articles supplied from thence were intended for spoon diets only, and could only be obtained by a requisition signed and countersigned; a great number of requisitions were sent in to Miss Nightingale's extra diet kitchen, but very far short of the number required. That this was so will appear from the following fact—the surgeons would constantly give us *verbal* permission to give a man nourishment or stimulants. We never for an instant thought of giving anything without this permission (I mean the ladies and Sisters of Mercy, not the hired nurses, who in this as in many other matters often could not be trusted).

We well knew that a man may apparently be sinking for want of food or stimulants, while his medical attendant would know it was the very worst thing for him; but when we received this verbal permission, we had no means of getting anything for the patients. We used to receive such orders as these:

"No. 1, give him anything you like. No. 2, he may have anything he can fancy. No. 3, keep him up as much as possible," and so on. Drinks for the fever patients were allowed in quantities could we only have had the materials to make them with. We could not get the assistant-surgeons to write out the number of requisitions which were necessary in order to procure these materials. At last, some of us persuaded one or two of our surgeons to write a requisition for dry stores; that is, for tins of preserved beef-tea, and for lemons and sugar to make lemonade. This was at first most successful. Many of the assistant-surgeons gladly accepted anything we prepared for the men. One difficulty only remained, *i.e.,* hot water. It was of course necessary to make the beef-tea, and also for the lemonade, as the water was so unwholesome it could not be used without boiling. We contrived to boil water in small quantities on the stoves in the corridors and wards. It was a slow process, but still we succeeded.

The orderlies seemed roused from the state of apathy into which the distress around and the apparent impossibility of getting anything for the patients had thrown them, and they assisted us in every possible way. Some of the orderlies looked with eager eyes on us as we carried round the small quantities of beef tea, for it was of course only to the patients belonging to the surgeons who wrote the requisitions that we could give the articles. One night a lady and her nurse were going round with some beef tea, when an orderly came up, and in a tone of entreaty pointed to a poor man. He was very bad, said he, "and some of that stuff would do him good, and the doctor said he might have anything he could fancy." The nurse turned round quick upon him.

"Orderly!"

"Yes, nurse!"

"What's the use of your asking impossibilities? You know very well that we can't give this beef-tea to your men. You must get your doctor to write a requisition for a tin of beef-tea!"

"Oh, very well, nurse," said the orderly, "I will."

"But that is not all," replied she; "at the same time get him to write a requisition for hot water!"

Our plan of thus helping the men was put a stop to by an order from Dr. Cumming, the inspector-general, that no cooking was to be done in the wards, and thus our only means of assisting the men was ended.

We seldom dressed the wounds, as there were dressers who performed this office, and the greater number of our patients were cases of fever and dysentery, who needed constant attention and nourishment, frequently administered in small quantities, and this we were now not suffered to give. All the diets not issued from Miss Nightingale's kitchen were of such a bad quality, and so wretchedly cooked, that the men often could not eat them. After a man had been put on half or even full diet, the surgeons were often obliged to return him to spoon diet from his not being able to eat the meat.

It was very hard work after Dr. Cumming's order had been issued to pace the corridor and hear perhaps the low voice of a fever patient, "Give me a drink for the love of God," and have none to give—for water we dared not give to any; or to see the look of disappointment on the faces of those to whom we had been accustomed to give the beef tea. The assistant-surgeons were very sorry, they said, for the alteration, but they had no power to help it— their duty was only to obey.

On one occasion an assistant-surgeon told us that Dr. Cumming had threatened to arrest him for having allowed a man too many extras on the diet roll. Amid all the confusion and distress of Scutari hospital, military discipline was never lost sight of, and an infringement of one of its smallest observances was worse than letting twenty men die from neglect.

The General Hospital, Scutari, stands about a mile from the Barrack Hospital; it is built close to the cliff, and commands a most beautiful view of Constantinople and the Sea of Marmora. It is a very fine building, not so large as the Barrack, and it holds with ease one thousand men, allowing room for doctors, chaplains, nurses, &c. The nurses at the General Hospital were then superintended by Miss Smythe, who shortly afterwards went to Koulali, and assisting her were three of Miss Sellon's Sisters, one lady, five nuns of the community called the "Kinsale Nuns," and I think about ten nurses. The ladies had a diet kitchen, and the routine was the same as at the Barrack Hospital.

When we went out for a walk it was generally to this hospital, or to the cliff around it. On one side of the General Hospital is the British burying ground, a spot which we could never visit without emotion, for there rested, oh! how many of England's noble sons! Whenever we went, they were digging graves, for from fifty to seventy a day were interred. Once we saw the cart loaded with the bodies coming slowly along, but we turned away, for the sight was too much to bear. The burying ground is beautifully situated, just on the edge of the cliff—the sea lies spread before it.

On one side in the distance lies Constantinople; on the opposite shore, far beyond where the eye can reach, stretches the great cemetery of the Turks, thickly studded with cypresses, and the strange tombstones of various colours, with their different devices, the turban, the broken lily, and other heathen emblems. Dark and gloomy looks the vast cemetery whither the Turk prays to be borne, that, when European Turkey shall become the property of the Christian, his bones may rest with his fathers.

Brightly in the open sunshine under no dark cypress' shade rest Britain's loved and lost. Here and there a stone or wooden cross marks in Whose name and in what hope we laid them down. The blue waves sparkle beneath their resting-place; the birds sing sweetly over their graves; the grass grows green over the mound, and in their countrypeople's hearts the spot must ever be sacred.

Returning from our walk over the wide plain which lies between the two hospitals, one's heart was weighed down by the thought of that mighty mass of suffering inside those walls, the sounds of which, though unheard by men, went up to the ear of Heaven. The thought of its immensity and apparent hopelessness was oppressive beyond description. All that was done for relief seemed but a drop in the ocean, and ere things could get to rights, or order be restored, how many hundreds of precious lives would have passed away!

Day succeeded day with little variation, and suffering and agony went on and on, and the angel of death stayed not his hand, but went swiftly day and night through those corridors and wards and took hundreds with him as he passed. In the morning when we entered our wards sad it was to see the numbers of empty beds.

In B corridor at one time were two cases of fever in a very bad state. The orderly attending them was a brute; he never did anything for them unless desired by the surgeon or nurse, and all the poor creatures did in the wildness of their delirium he treated as if it was done on purpose. He declared that they *would* tear the wet rags from their heads, and it was no use to put them on again, and he never replaced them unless we obliged him; he used to put down their food by their sides, just as if they were strong and sensible, and able to help themselves, instead of the poor hands lying helpless by their sides, or clutching and picking the bed clothes, the unerring sign to those who know sickness well that their days on earth were numbered.

Poor fellows! their passage through the valley of the shadow of death was hard indeed. They lingered many days. Among so very many others we could not give them much time. One day passing by their beds I saw one of them was near death. I was obliged to go to our quarters on an errand for another patient. I made all possible haste, and in a quarter of an hour returned to the bed of death, but the bed was vacant—he had died, been wrapped in his blanket, and carried away to the dead house—the other died that night.

Death indeed became familiar to us as the ordinary events of life. Among one thousand five hundred sick committed to the care of three women, it was impossible to attend to the greater number, and it was grievous to be obliged to pass by so many sick on whom we longed to wait—cases like some of spotted fever in A corridor—and see the poor hands grasping the sheets, and the sufferer in his delirium refusing the medicine on which his life hung.

The want of clean linen was bitterly felt at that time in Scutari. How it was issued from the stores was a mystery no one could ever unravel. If things were sent to be washed, they never returned, and there was not the slightest order or regularity in the issue of linen, either sheets or shirts. Towels and pocket-handkerchiefs were both considered unnecessary luxuries for the soldiers, and could be obtained only from Miss Nightingale's free-gift store, and, generally speaking, only from them could flannel shirts be had. Orderlies thought nothing of taking off a soiled flannel from a man and giving him a clean cotton in exchange.

Confusion, indeed, so prevailed in all quarters at that unhappy time, that though quantities of things were sent to Scutari but few ever reached the sufferers for whom they were destined. Every ship that came in brought to Miss Nightingale large packages of every imaginable article of wearing apparel; great numbers of bales of old linen and lint also arrived, and these last were quite useless, as both were amply supplied from the medical stores of the hospital.

The packages were unpacked and put into Miss Nightingale's free-gift store, which was a large shed outside the hospital. It was impossible for Miss Nightingale, with her numerous and arduous avocations, to find time even to look at them; no one had the regular charge of them; nurses and sometimes ladies when they had time went to assist at the endless task of putting them to rights.

There was another store inside the hospital, which was under the charge of the Superioress of the Sisters of Mercy; this store was kept in beautiful order, but was quite full. From neither of these stores of Miss Nightingale could anything be procured but on the same plan as the diets, *i.e.*, a doctor's requisition signed and countersigned. It was even more impossible to get these than the others for diets, from a feeling amongst the surgeons that clothing for the men ought to have come from Government stores, and not liking fully to acknowledge the gross neglect of the purveying department. So, we only saw how miserably the men were off, and were obliged to leave them so.

It was a common thing to find men with sheets and shirts unchanged for weeks. I have opened the collar of a patient's shirt and found it literally lined with vermin. It was common to find men covered with sores from lying in one position on the hard straw beds and coarse sheets, and there were no pillows to put under them. Pillows were unknown to the Government stores, and we could not get requisitions for them from Miss Nightingale's free gift store. The only exceptions to this rule were that some articles which were given to the nurses they gave away to the patients. Mrs. Bracebridge gave away numbers of things from the free gift store, chiefly to those who assisted in the unpacking of them. By this means we sometimes gained possession of shirts, or pocket handkerchiefs, or towels, and they were much prized by the men.

A great deal of sickness prevailed among ourselves; two nurses at this time were lying ill with fever, one not expected to live; two out of the five nuns were in the same state—they both lay for days at the point of death, but ultimately recovered. During the whole of their illness, they remained in the room where the three other Sisters slept and ate. There was no infirmary to remove the sick ladies to. The sick nurses were taken to a room outside the hospital. Of those among ladies and nurses not ill with fever many were laid up for a day or two at a time from over fatigue and want of proper food.

Our life was a laborious one; we had to sweep our own room, make our beds, wash up our dishes, &c., and fetch our meals from the kitchen below. We went to our wards at nine, returned at two, went again at three (unless we went out for a walk, which we had permission to do at this hour), returned at half-past five to tea, then to the wards again till half-past nine, and often again for an hour to our special cases. We had prayers read by Mr. Bracebridge at eight in the morning, and at nine at night one of the chaplains came; but at that time, they were often prevented from press of work.

We suffered greatly from want of proper food. Our diet consisted of the coarse sour bread of the country, tea without milk, butter so rancid we could not touch it, and very bad meat and porter; and at night a glass of wine or brandy. It was an effort even to those in health to sit down to our meals; we forced the food down as a duty, but some of the ladies became so weak and ill they really could not touch it.

For one in particular we tried to get a little milk or an egg, but both these articles were scarce; a small quantity of both was taken into Miss Nightingale's and Mr. and Mrs. Bracebridge's rooms, but could not be furnished to the rest of the party. Occasionally Miss Nightingale kindly sent some light dish from her own table to the sick ladies. The nuns took all their meals in their own apartments, the nurses in theirs, the ladies in theirs: Miss Nightingale and Mr. and Mrs. Bracebridge in their own apartment.

The quantity of vermin in the wards was past conception; the men's clothes and beds swarmed with them, so did every room in the hospital. Our clothes had their full share, and the misery they caused us was very great: we never slept more than an hour at a time because of them. We much rejoiced, on reaching Scutari, to find plenty of blankets, which we never had at Therapia, and the want of which there we had been feeling in the cold winter nights; but when we found that the surface of the blanket was closely dotted with tiny black spots, our joy somewhat diminished. The poor men felt this very much, but of course without clean linen it could not be helped.

People have often spoken of the patience, courage, and endurance of the sick in English hospitals, but they have only pain to endure, and doctors are busy to alleviate this, and careful to give them all necessary comforts. It was in the Eastern hospitals that the true heroism of patient courage was pre-eminently displayed. We have attended many hundreds of the sick of the British Army suffering under every form of disease—the weary wasting of low typhus fever or dysentery, or the agony of frostbite—and they were surrounded by every accumulation of misery.

For the fevered lips was there no cooling drink; for the sinking frame no strengthening food; for the sore limb no soft pillow; for many no watchful hands to help; but never did we hear a murmur pass those lips. We have seen the brave and strong man laid low; have seen him watch death coming, and meet it calmly, for he died in doing his duty. Oh! that they who speak harshly of the British soldier had been with those whose privilege it was to nurse him—had witnessed that wonderful spectacle of the woe of the winter of 1854 and—55—had seen the obedience to orders, the respectful gratitude, the noble qualities there displayed!

Often did our hearts burn within us as we passed along, as we heard the thanks and blessings poured upon those who were doing oh! so miserably little for so great affliction; or as we knelt by the dying to hear his last request to write home and tell them all about him; or as we watched the death struggle, and saw one noble heart after another cease to beat.

The sick came in almost daily, so that the beds which death had emptied during the night were sure to be filled again in the course of the day. Sad it was to see the sick coming in, the orderlies putting down the stretchers and looking round in despair for a bed to lay the poor sufferer on: a low moan was the only evidence of the torture he was enduring, or how he longed to be laid in any place where he could die in peace. Then again, they hastily raised the stretcher on their shoulder, giving frequent jerks to the agonised frame, and turned down another corridor in search of a bed. We whispered to ourselves:

Patience, deeply-suffering ones, all is not forgotten, every drop in this most bitter cup is portioned out for you, and as you drink it will be treasured up in heaven. You have followed bravely an earthly captain to victory through wounds and over dying comrades, follow now the Great Captain of your salvation through the dark valley.

Sickness is sad at all times—sad is it to languish and suffer on our soft English beds, with skilful physicians full of anxiety, with tender nurses and loving friends, with every comfort earth can give; but only those who saw can enter into the dreariness of those sick beds. It was so sad to see them die one after another—we learned to love them so—ever ringing in our ears seemed the anxious hopes and prayers of the fond hearts in England.

The mother's only stay was there, or the loved husband or brother, and they were dying, not in the glory of the battlefield, but in these dreary corridors. They who had fought so bravely suffered so nobly; they who, if they had lived, would have been honoured by a nation's gratitude—they were passing away by hundreds—no name would mark their graves, and they would, save in the loving hearts of home, be soon forgotten.

No, not forgotten either. Surely when the tale of that memorable winter shall be told, when future generations shall hear how they stormed at Alma, charged at Balaclava, and held their ground at Inkermann, how they resolutely waited before the walls of Sebastopol, till at length the gallantly defended city yielded to her dauntless foes England will not forget those who shed their blood for her sake, though no glory hovered round their death-bed, save a ray from His glory who first taught us to be "*obedient unto death.*" Sad it was to hear the tales they would tell, such mere boys as some of them were, how they had enlisted in a moment of folly and bitterly regretted it, or to listen to their long accounts of friends at home; how they would describe every little incident relating to them as if it were engraven on their hearts.

Very often we wrote letters home for them from their dictation; we sat on their beds to do it, for there were no other seats of any kind. It often struck us the eagerness with which they accepted our offer to write a letter for any of them—they hardly ever asked us to do so—they seemed to be so resigned to everything, that it was quite a surprise to them to be able to have a sheet of paper and an envelope placed at their disposal, still more a friend's hand to write for them; and then they were so full of solicitude "Were we not too tired to do it? or was it not uncomfortable sitting on that there bed?"

CHAPTER 5

Koulali

After a fortnight had been spent among these scenes, a change occurred in the nursing arrangements. Miss Stanley at Koulali was in great want of additional hands, as she found her staff inefficient to the work of the hospitals of Koulali, and requested help from Miss Nightingale. Miss N. gave leave to all the ladies at Scutari to volunteer for Koulali. Miss Smythe and myself did so, and another lady followed us in a few days.

Koulali is about five miles north of Scutari. I once went there from Scutari in a Turkish carriage; the drive was for some distance through the Turkish cemetery, which, as I said before, extends for miles round Scutari. There are no roads in Turkey worthy of the name, nor have the carriages any springs; between these two misfortunes one runs a chance of being jolted to death. Certainly, I never expected to reach Koulali with whole bones, and firmly determined as it was my first drive in a Turkish carriage it should be my last.

Koulali barracks are built on the banks of the Bosphorus, a few yards from the quay; the depth of water allows steamers to come alongside the quay, therefore its facility for landing the sick is very great. The hospital is a square red building three storeys high in front, very much smaller than Scutari, but a large building nevertheless. The principal entrance is raised a few feet from the quay, ascending which you pass under the archway into the barrack-yard. Apartments are built over the archway, called the *Sultan's* apartments, at that time occupied by the *commandant*, chaplains, and medical officers. Standing under the archway, to the right and left, were the wards, which extended more than halfway round the square, two storeys high. Opposite were stables, which were then about to be made into wards.

The wards were of a very peculiar construction, a long corridor, with a gallery over it; the doors of almost all open upon the different entrances of the hospital, which all have archways. This made the wards seem like separate buildings, though on the upper storey, by passing through rooms, one can walk from one end of the hospital to the other, only descending at the different entrances. The three entrances were all guarded by sentries.

Built in continuation of the hospital on the quay are more rooms and stables, occupied by the Turkish soldiers; beyond this comes the riding-school, which was just then converted into the convalescent hospital: a most delightful one it made. It was divided into twelve wards, partitioned off by woodwork about eleven feet high; the roof was high with open beams. This hospital was well warmed and ventilated; there was an apartment for the surgeon in charge—and the surgery and kitchen were built off.

The situation was delightful, as all those able to walk could get outside the hospital and catch the fresh breeze from the sea. Hills rose immediately around Koulali; it was literally shut in on all sides between hills and water. Great fears were entertained at that time that in the heat of summer this would render it unhealthy; these fears were, however, happily never realised. On the first hill above the Barrack Hospital, on the Scutari side, was built the General Hospital.

The Turks always appear to build an hospital close to their barracks. Both buildings were now British hospitals. We distinguished them as Barrack and General hospitals, or sometimes upper and lower. It was a good climb up the hill to the General Hospital, but one was rewarded by the fresh air and lovely view.

The General Hospital was built on the plan of Scutari—two stories high, corridor running round, and wards out of them. It held with comfort two hundred and fifty men, with apartments for medical officers and nurses. Of course, at that time many more were obliged to be accommodated. At the upper hospital apartments were provided for the Catholic Sisters of Mercy, some of whom came down to nurse in wards at the barrack hospitals, while a few ladies and nurses went up to help the rest of the Sisters in the General Hospital.

Our apartments were in one corner of the lower hospital, for at each corner there was a small corridor, with half-a-dozen small rooms opening out of it. Among these rooms there was a very small kitchen, which, however, we contrived to make our extra diet kitchen. A dark closet formed our store-room. There was one large kitchen for the general use, where the meat for the full and half diets was cooked; but the hospital was so crowded, the cookery arrangements so wretched, that our aid in cooking the spoon diets was gladly accepted by the doctors.

In the hospitals of Koulali at that time were very few wounded. The wounded of Alma and Inkermann had either recovered or died. It was the sick from the trenches who poured down upon us. Fever, dysentery, diarrhoea, and frost-bite were our four principal diseases, and the sufferers were those who, having struggled with disease to the last, came down with their constitutions broken and needing careful nursing. We were received and treated from first to last with the utmost cordiality, courtesy, and kindness by the army surgeons.

Dr. Tice was then principal medical officer, succeeded shortly after by Dr. Humphrey. The principal medical officer was of course the one under whose immediate orders we were placed. By these gentlemen we were treated with uniform kindness; they instructed us in what way we could be most useful, and always spoke warmly of the assistance we rendered them.

The wards of Koulali hospital were classified: No. 2, surgical; No. 3, fever; No. 4, dysentery; No. 5, diarrhoea; No. 6, dysentery. Every ward was full. We had then one thousand men, with very few exceptions all confined to bed, and hardly a case not a most serious one. Our duties were to accompany the surgeon round the wards to receive his orders for the day, then attending to the food and medicine, seeing to the linen, and feeding those too weak to feed themselves. (This is one instance where nurses are wanted to carry out the surgeon's orders. He may order a man medicine, wine, and nourishment, and the article he furnished, and then the orderly sets it down by the patient's side and thinks no more about it, whilst the patient is perhaps weaker than an infant, or unconscious of what he is doing.) Then came writing letters, procuring books for those a little better and able to read—newspapers were always precious, but at that time an untold boon.

Our plan was to receive the surgeon's *verbal* orders for the men's food, and if there was any difficulty about the requisitions, or when the requisitions were procured having them honoured by the purveyor, we supplied them out of our own kitchen. The doctors constantly left numbers of cases in our charge to be fed as we thought best. Whenever a verbal order was given, the lady or Sister wrote her own requisition on the ladies' diet-kitchen and it was immediately attended to, as far as our Free Gift's Store would allow.

In the evenings the surgeons visited their wards; then came the night-drinks' distribution, sorely needed by all, for thirst was acutely felt by the frostbitten and dysentery as well as the fever patients. Late at night, very weary, we sought our quarters. Gladly would we have undertaken night work, but our numbers were far from adequate for the labour of the day. All had a far larger portion than was commensurate to their strength, and only by God's especial help did we keep up at all.

Almost immediately on our arrival two of our party, being ill, were removed to the *Hotel des Croissants,* Buyukdere, twelve miles down the Bosphorus, on the European side. The next day they sickened with fever. One paid nurse accompanied them. One of the nuns fell ill with fever the following day, so our number was reduced to eighteen for both hospitals.

The same day the Misses —— left; we had hardly seen them off in a *caique* when an alarm that our quarter was on fire burst upon our ears. It proceeded from the kitchen, and it was discovered that the flue of the chimney had been so built that if it got heated it must catch fire.

This was a common specimen of Turkish building. In five minutes, the engineer officer and his men were on the spot, and by their prompt and vigorous efforts the fire, which was now bursting out, was arrested. Two engines played for five hours before danger was over, and then what a scene! The kitchen unroofed, the wall of one bedroom broken in, and the corridor a floating mass of mud, water, and stones—another room so stuffed with furniture we could not move.

The frost was just beginning to set in. We stood in the barrack-yard watching the devastation with resignation, and wondering where we should sleep that night. We did not wonder long, for the officers and chaplains with ready kindness offered us the choice of their quarters. We accepted the principal room in the *Sultan's* quarters, which the *commandant* vacated for our use; two of the bedrooms in the old quarters were sufficiently habitable to accommodate the three nurses.

From this time the whole party of ladies ate, drank, and slept in one apartment. We felt that Miss Stanley who filled so arduous and responsible a position needed a separate room and more tempting food than at that time fell to our lot; but although her health suffered from these causes, she resolutely refused to have any luxuries or comforts in which all those about her could not partake.

To add to our troubles, the next day one of the three nurses sickened with fever. Of course, each separate case of fever among ourselves not only caused the loss of the invalid from the nursing staff, but the principal, if not the whole, services of another to attend upon her.

Chapter 6

Arrival of Irish Soldiers at the Hospital

How were we to supply our "extra diet" kitchen, how prepare the food on which so many depended? The erection of a shed in the barrack-yard was immediately set on foot; but it took ten days ere we gained possession of it, and our only resource was three or four small charcoal brasiers. Charcoal always drawing so much more quickly in the open air, we placed them in the barrack-yard.

"Misfortunes never come singly;" so we thought when John, the soldier cook, fell sick and had to go into the fever ward. Then the thaw came, and the yard was a mass of snow and black mud, and then it alternately froze and thawed, making our weary hours in the barrack-yard seem long indeed. Our cook ill, we cooked for ourselves, our only staff being Henry, a sailor lad, and the Greeks, who had not the slightest conscience as to appropriating anything that pleased them; serious indeed was our loss if they did, for our "free gift" store was very scanty, and of course we could only draw the exact quantity allowed by the diet roll, so that an egg once lost was not easily replaced; an ounce of arrowroot or sugar was worth more than its weight in gold, while a saucepan to boil it in, or a spoon to stir it with, was guarded by its fortunate possessors with a dragon-like vigilance.

After ten days we gained possession of a kitchen, which was in two divisions, one was in the *Sultan's* quarters, the other the shed in the yard; John recovered and took charge of the first, Henry of the shed; part of the cookery was carried on in one, and the rest in the other. Great joy was caused by a gift of Lady Stratford de Redcliffe of a large stove for charcoal, upon which we could fry as well as boil. Lady Stratford had given the stove some time before but it could not be used till it could be placed in a kitchen.

Our quarters which had been burned were now refitted, and we should have returned thither had not the officers most kindly insisted upon making the exchange, thus relinquishing the best rooms to our use; namely, four rooms in the *Sultan's* quarters, of which one we used ourselves, one as an infirmary, and two were occupied by the nurses. Dr. and Mrs. Tice and the two Church of England chaplains occupied the remainder of the rooms on the left side of the archway. The *bey* who commanded the Turkish troops lived on the right side; and we had a room to keep our stores in instead of a dark closet.

By slow and strenuous efforts, we gradually improved the state of the kitchen. We were able by means of our stove to fry a small quantity of chops. In one of the boilers in our kitchen shed we boiled fowls, and then cut them in half for the patients. Another boiler contained water for arrowroot; everything was on the roughest scale the orderlies brought large cans or wooden buckets, put their arrowroot and cold water into them, and stirred it up with a bit of stick, then Henry dispensed the boiling water, and of course the orderlies fought who should get it first.

The lady in charge put in the wine, and the arrowroot was carried to the Sister or lady in charge of each ward, and dispensed to the men. Persons accustomed to make the delicate food for some dear invalid, or who have watched the beautiful order of the kitchen of a London hospital, will smile at our extra diets for the sick; nevertheless they were gladly received by the poor sufferers, who thought them an improvement upon *nothing*.

But the labour of life was lemonade. The patients suffered much from thirst, and those who were ordered lemonade were very numerous. The sight of a lemon squeezer (no such article could be furnished from the stores) would have been very gratifying, the cutting and squeezing were so long and tiresome. We employed the Greeks about it, but their help was not to be depended on; sometimes they would work, at others suddenly depart for hours; and they would, moreover, pocket lemons, or other things to any extent.

Besides, all the Greeks in Government employ went home at sunset; and the chief call for lemonade was in the evenings. One evening a lady made a large pailful, and went into the "dark closet" for sugar; she put it into the lemonade, stirred it up and tasted it to see if all was right, but it was salt she had put in instead of sugar; and wearily did she set about the task of making more; cut more lemons, and get more water—all the water came from a tank at the extreme end of the barrack yard, and had to be fetched by Greeks, who took an enormous time about it, so that water became very precious.

Our difficulties daily increased; the two sick ladies at Buyukdere were so alarmingly ill that the surgeon attending them required another nurse. We sent one of the hired nurses, but she returned the next day, having been found by the surgeon in a state of dead intoxication in the room of one of the ladies, then trembling between life and death; of course, the nurse had to be sent home. One of the ladies of our party went to nurse the two others; another, whose duty it was, in addition to the care of her ward, to superintend the kitchen department, was suffering so from inflammation and weakness as to be often unable to leave her bed for a day or more.

The light conduct of another of the hired nurses, even at this time of distress, obliged her dismissal. The one who had been intoxicated was to accompany a lady to Scutari, from thence to take her passage to England. She went down quite quietly to the water's edge, put one foot into the *caique* in which the lady was sitting, and then jumped into the water, running the narrowest chance of upsetting the boat, in which case the lady must have been lost, as the strength of the current was fearful; the unfortunate woman was dragged out, and immediately went into what was apparently an epileptic fit.

She was carried to her bed, on which she would not lie, but broke the windows, tore the matting from the floor and her hair from her head. Poor woman! she had before that openly avowed her belief that there was no God! After some days she recovered, was sent home, and, I believe, is now a nurse in a London hospital. Such and many similar tales could be told of those who came from and returned to nurse the poor of England.

March opened with variations of cold and days of spring-like loveliness. Once, as a great event, we took a walk to the Turkish cemetery. The lady superintendent, fearing our health would completely give way, desired us to do so—how we enjoyed the fresh air and lovely view after our long confinement to the wards!

Our next trouble was the sickening with fever of the third lady who had gone to nurse the two others at Buyukdere, and also of the nurse who had been sent to assist her. There were now at Buyukdere four in bed; the two first out of immediate danger, but in a most precarious state. Miss Nightingale kindly sent a nurse from Scutari, for from our staff we knew not how to spare one.

It was a sad sight to see these three ladies lying in a foreign hotel, far from friends and home, and suffering under a deadly disease, their companions unable to be with them; but a merciful Father raised up help as it was needed. One of the surgeons of the naval hospital, Therapia (three miles from Buyukdere), attended them all through their illness—twice a day, sometimes oftener, did he come from his own arduous duties to their bedsides; he was not only physician, but, as they afterwards expressed it, "father and brother his kindness was beyond words to express. The ladies belonging to the naval hospital also came forward with Sisterly kindness in this time of distress. One who had herself risen from a bed of sickness took her turn to watch at night by the bedside of those who were strangers to her.

At Koulali the work did not abate; as quickly as we sent home convalescents to England, so did others begin to pour in from the camp. The Irish soldiers now came down in shoals. We suppose this was caused by their constitutions being more inured to hardships than the English, and their having in consequence held out longer, although now worn out.

Oh! what grievous scenes was our daily life now passed among! The cases of frost-bite exceeded in horror all one had ever imagined. Dressing wounds was not our business; there were "dressers" who fulfilled this office; when the frost-bite had extended so far up the foot that it could not be stopped, amputation was the only means of saving life, and it even was but a chance, for their constitutions were so broken that many were unable to rally from the shock. At this time in the surgical ward were three men just in this state, Fitzgerald, Flack, and Cooney.

Fitzgerald had lost a foot, so had the two others, and some of the toes of the remaining foot. Cooney was about eighteen or nineteen; he was an Irish Catholic. Poor fellow! he suffered so much from being obliged to lie in one position that he was covered with sores. He was so thin his bones seemed almost coming through his skin; and his state was such that not even an orderly was allowed to turn him from one side to another; but the surgeon had to do it himself, and Dr. Temple most tenderly did it for him. Dr. Temple was one who almost lived in his ward, who thought no trouble too much, no time too long, to be devoted to his men.

Severe things have been said of the medical department of the army; and its members were, apparently, so despised that their work was taken from them in some measure, and put into the hands of civilians. No doubt some of the heads of the department who had grown old under the old system of military hospitals, and were unable to realise the necessity of a prompt and immediate change, were obstinate and hard-hearted.

No doubt among such a large body of men many young and careless ones, unfitted for the awfully responsible charge then placed in their hands, were to be found; but in condemning such the merits of others should not be overlooked. Most ungrateful were it if the nurses should omit recording their experience of the much dreaded "army surgeons." So misrepresented had this class of men been that it was with far more fear of them than of the horrors of hospital life that the ladies entered the hospital. They were told to expect rebuffs, discouragements, and even insult. During a year's residence among them the writer and all her companions never experienced from an army surgeon other than assistance, encouragement, and gentlemanly treatment, and from many of them the most cordial kindness.

The tenacity of life in poor Cooney was wonderful; day after day, night after night, he lived and suffered on; growing weaker and weaker. How his piteous moans went through the hearts of his attendants, how terrible was it to watch the distortion of agony on his young face. Poor boy! he was very patient, and he said he knew "it was best for him, or the good God would not send him such suffering, and his trust was in Him, and he did try to be patient." We used to tempt him with the best of the little at our disposal, for Dr. Temple ordered him anything he could fancy.

At length eggs, beat up with wine, were the only thing he could swallow, and until ten minutes before his death his nurse fed him with this. Death came at last, and he passed away as a child falls asleep, and with an intense relief did his attendants watch the calm, peaceful look on those features so long tortured with agony. One did not gaze long; in half-an-hour (and that was longer than usual) he was wrapped in his blanket, and carried to the dead-house.

Then there was poor Flack; he suffered too, we thought, the extent of human suffering. He was covered with sores, one foot off, and two toes of the other; he was ordered anything he liked, but in vain: he was in too much pain to eat, he "cared for nothin'—nothin' would save him." One day he said, "ell ye what I could eat—a bit of apple-pudding!" But, oh dear! we thought, how was it to be got? how get the flour and the apples? and how get it boiled? However, it was made, but he could hardly touch it, though he insisted on its being set down by his side. Another man had the same fancy, and he declared it had "done him more good than all the physic." Poor Flack died one night—quite quietly, they told us.

Fitzgerald, we watched by many a time, expecting to see him die; he looked just like a corpse; his strength was utterly gone. Among so many interesting cases he was one distinguished from all others, not only by his patience, but his cheerfulness. He was an Irishman all over, always merry, and making the best of everything; his gratitude for being waited upon was great. Even when apparently in a dying state he would look up into our faces and smile. He lingered on, his doctors having no hope of his recovery; it seemed impossible he could rally from such a shock.

However, he did; his improvement at first was very gradual, but three months afterwards we had the satisfaction of seeing him leave the hospital for England, though of course a cripple still as stout and rosy as one could wish to see; his face quite radiant with happiness at the thought of going back to "ould Ireland." Each ward contained at that time sixty beds, and to give an idea how crowded we were it is enough to say that the number was afterwards reduced to thirty. Each patient lay on a low trestle bed, raised a few inches from the ground.

The news of the death of the Emperor of Russia came upon us with startling effect. Miss Stanley went through the wards and announced it to the men.

"Long life to ye!" said many of the Irish, in a tone of congratulation, as though we had been the instruments of his death. "It is better than a month's pay!" said another, and "God be praised!" cried many a sufferer.

It was curious enough that the day of the death of the emperor was signalised by an earthquake of a very violent nature. That scene will never be forgotten by those who witnessed it. It occurred about three o'clock in the afternoon. The day before a heavy mist hung over the Bosphorus—a very unusual thing for Turkey. The hospital was shaken most violently; an instant rush was made by the nurses for the barrack-yard. Many of the poor patients jumped out of their beds, and, forgetting their sufferings in their terror, ran down the wards with fearful cries, and when the immediate excitement was over were unable to return to their beds without assistance. The clocks fell from the walls, and innumerable articles rolled about in great confusion. The extraordinary costumes of the patients and their extreme terror made the scene, awful as it was, almost ludicrous.

The lower division of the fever ward was occupied by Russian prisoners—such of them as were too ill to be removed when the hospital was given up to the British. They were attended by our surgeons, and we occasionally sent cocoa to them, but were forbidden by Lord William Paulet to visit them. It has before been remarked that the upper division of each ward was like a gallery with open palings. One of our patients in a fit of delirium jumped over these palings into the ward below, and falling upon one of the poor patients broke his collar-bone. The Russian never could be induced to believe but that it was done on purpose.

The cases of delirium among the poor patients were very trying. I remember one of the orderlies calling upon me to persuade a man to go to bed; his manner and tone were those of a man completely in his senses, but calmly and earnestly he assured me that he had committed the most horrible crimes, that justice was about to overtake him, and that it was useless for him to go to bed, as he was about to be plunged into a dark dungeon. He continued in this state for days, and could never be kept in bed except by force; and one day he leaped over the palings into the ward below and was killed on the spot.

One poor patient among the frost-bitten attracted my attention by his constant refusal to take any sort of food, or to receive any kind of comfort that was offered to him. For a long time, he would not speak, but one day, on my offering to write home for him, he burst into tears and told me his history. He had been attacked by frost-bite in the camp, and had been placed on a mule to go to Balaclava, there to embark for Koulali. The mule on which he rode was fastened to another, carrying baggage, which slipped and fell upon him. None of the party conducting the sick possessed so much as a knife to cut the straps which connected the two mules, and so for many minutes the mule lay upon him till a sailor, accidentally coming by, released him from his dreadful position.

He was brought to Koulali hospital and treated for frost-bite, but when in a fair way of recovery from this, and with the prospect of coming home invalided, it was discovered that he had sustained a severe internal injury, from which there was but slight hope of his recovery, and the disappointment seemed to make his cup of sorrow run over, and he lay there in utter despair, not caring how soon death might release him. He was a member of the Church of England and had been religiously brought up and was one of the many who had enlisted in a moment of folly, and afterwards bitterly lamented his rash step.

We became great friends from that day. He grew more cheerful, and willingly took whatever I wished him, and his gratitude was unbounded. He, however, became much better, but was then seized with typhus fever. He managed to rally through this also, and was able to walk to church that night he was seized with inflammation and died two days afterwards.

These cases I insert as specimens of the kind then passing under our hands. The memory of each lady and Sister of Mercy would supply many such. Our occupations were so overwhelming that those working in the Barrack Hospital had not time even to visit the General Hospital, so that no more can be said than that this hospital proceeded on the same routine as the Barrack Hospital. The plan was for both hospitals to be served by Sisters, ladies, and nurses, but of the two latter classes the ladies were ill, and the nurses either the same or dismissed for immoral conduct.

The whole burden, therefore, fell upon the Sisters, who admirably fulfilled their duties, giving great satisfaction to the Lady Superintendent and the medical officers. It would be only repetition to describe their work at this juncture, as it was like that executed by the ladies and Sisters in the Barrack Hospital.

CHAPTER 6

Unwearied Zeal of the Sisters of Mercy

Extraordinary were the scenes our one room would witness in the course of the day. The successive knocks at the door would "bring a wild-looking Greek with a message, a grave Turk with another, a Scotch orderly, our Hungarian servant, his German wife, officers, French and Italian servants, an Irish nun, and an English lady."

On one occasion an orderly answered a lady impertinently in the ward, not choosing to attend to her directions for the patients' comfort. It was necessary to show the orderlies that we were instructed by the surgeons to carry out their orders, and, accordingly, when the medical officer in charge came his evening rounds, the lady reported the circumstance to him. We thought he would rebuke the man, and there would be an end of it. "Send him to the guardroom!" was the instant order. We were sorry, but of course thought the affair must end here.

Next morning a tall corporal appeared at our room door demanding the lady's attendance before the *commandant*. He did not say what it was for, and she was quite alarmed and went in evident terror to the extreme amusement of her companions. The *commandant* received her with his usual courtesy, and assured her that he was determined no instance of disrespect or disobedience to the orders of the ladies should be suffered among the orderlies, and therefore he only wanted her evidence to dismiss the man from his post of orderly. As the lady passed from the "order room," through the line of soldiers on guard, she firmly determined that the orderlies must behave *very* badly indeed ere she would punish *herself* so again for their good.

One of the minor trials of life was our want of a female servant. With the severe pulls upon our time and strength, the labour of tending our own room was very great. One day we were standing over the brasiers, cooking in the yard, when a tall and remarkable-looking foreigner, speaking very broken English, suddenly stood beside us and began to make remarks upon the style of cooking, especially that of Henry, the sailor. Poor Henry's was certainly an original style, particularly in what he prepared for our own table. He always chose to think most of that branch of his business, and his delight was to send up *recherche* dishes in which grease was the largest ingredient.

The stranger informed us his name was Papafée; that he had a wife and child; that he was an Hungarian refugee; had been an officer in the Austrian service; had castles and untold riches in Hungary, but, having taken the side of his country and Kossuth, had lost them all, and was obliged to fly and earn his bread. His wife was a German, and could, he said, do household and needlework: as to himself, he could do everything according to his own account—he could "speak nine languages, write, keep accounts, shop, interpret, cook" in short, he was perfect.

Notwithstanding these perfections, as far as himself was concerned, we should have been unmindful of them; but we gladly engaged him for the sake of his wife, who, indeed, proved to us a treasure. Gentle, willing, and industrious, little Rosalie was a ray of comfort in our distress, though it was somewhat counterbalanced by her husband, who did everything we asked him with an air of infinite condescension, as if he were a monarch waiting on his subjects—to forget to ask him for everything before he went downstairs was an offence not easily forgiven. To want a spoon or glass more than he allowed would bring down a severe rebuke on our heads.

He used to favour us with his opinion of things in general; whenever we offended him, he would scold at us, not allowing our voices to be heard in self-defence, and, saying "It ees veri diificulte to please everybode!" would fling himself out of the room. It was, however, an amusement, and many a laugh did we have over his eccentricities.

Our invalids at Buyukdere still continued very ill, so did the Sister and nurse of our party. Our whole staff now consisted of nine Sisters, three ladies, and two nurses, and now Miss Smythe fell ill. She had been the stay of the lady party till now, never having suffered in the least from sickness: she had the charge of the fever ward, and her labours there were great and unremitting: I never saw a person more zealously devoted to her work. She, as well as the others, almost lived in her ward; her whole thought seemed to be for her patients—she fed them and waited upon them with most attentive care. She caught a violent cold so as to quite take away her voice.

We begged of her to stay at home and nurse; but if she had, no one could have taken her place in the fever ward, and leave her men she would not. She went and stayed all day as usual, and would come back at tea time looking: most worn and fatigued, and but with difficulty was persuaded to give up her evening rounds, which another undertook to attend to in addition to her own, while Miss Smythe went to bed.

After going round the long fever ward with night drinks, this lady was about to return home, when a poor man raised, himself up and said, "Is not that ere lady a coming here tonight?" She explained the reason of her absence. "But is not she a cooking something for me?" No, she was not. "Well," said he, lying down again with a resigned look, "I be *very* hungry." The lady went back to quarters and asked Miss Smythe. She said he was very weak and ordered by the medical officer anything he fancied. It was so late the kitchen was closed; however, we contrived to take him a little of Mr. Gamble's soup, and he was delighted, and said it was the "beautifulest" thing he had ever tasted.

For some days longer Miss Smythe struggled on, till at length she gave in of her own accord, and stayed in bed one day. On that day letters reached us announcing that in a fortnight or three weeks a staff of ladies and nurses for Koulali would arrive. The news raised our fainting spirits—poor Miss Smythe especially expressed much pleasure. It was the last conscious thing we heard her say. Next day fever came on, and delirium as usual followed. A very excellent nurse attended her, and most skilful surgeons; all that could be done for her was done, and though we knew her case was a most severe one, still we hoped on, for up to this time all the members of our staff attacked with fever had escaped death, though all had hung for days at its very point.

On the 27th of March the chaplain of the Church of England administered the Communion to her; she was partly conscious at the time. Throughout her illness she had always displayed great patience; but she seldom spoke, and was constantly delirious. All this day the doctors spoke very badly of her case, but still we hoped against hope.

March 28th I was in the act of distributing the dinners to the orderlies for their wards, when the news of her death was brought to me, and it fell like the shock of a sudden death; and yet, such was our strange life at that time, I could not leave my employment, but was obliged to count out mutton-chops and half fowls till the hospital was served, and then went upstairs to the room of death. She died without a sigh, and in a state of unconsciousness. She had suffered from a malignant form of typhus fever, and the surgeons said that interment the next day was absolutely necessary.

Next day she was buried; the coffin was covered with a white sheet, the orderlies of her ward carried her body up the steep path which led from the hospital to the graveyard. All the convalescents wished to follow, but the cold was thought too keen for them. Ourselves and the officers followed the coffin, and we laid her on the green hill-side far away from the old churchyards of England, but we felt the ground was in some sense sacred, from the noble and brave who rested there.

A sudden chill came on us as we stood around her grave; the sun was sinking below the horizon, and lighting up distant Constantinople, the blue Bosphorus, and dark hills with its last glow. On one side lay in shade the Turkish Cemetery, the sad token that we were in a stranger land.

It was with a lonely feeling we laid her there, far away from friends and home, yet we knew God and His angels were as near, perhaps even nearer, to the exiles. She was not forgotten in Koulali. Deep was the regret expressed by the patients in the fever wards at the sudden death of their kind attendant. Many tears were shed for her; they spoke of her with real affection, and treasured up every instance of her kindness and self-denial. We immediately placed a small wooden cross at the head of her grave, and one of the soldiers carved her initials on it. We put it there to mark the spot till we could learn the wishes of her relatives on the point.

At their desire her grave was afterwards covered with a stone monument, bearing simply the inscription of her name and date of her death. No word of praise follows, as thus it is ever meet the Christian should rest—he needs it not; for her the world's applause has passed away as shadows fleet before the sun. But we leave her in the humble hope that she will one day hear the words, "*Inasmuch as ye did it unto the least of these, ye did it unto Me.*"

Two days after the funeral Miss Stanley left for England. She had already, at Lady Stratford's earnest request, delayed her departure for some weeks. Her departure was deeply regretted by all, especially the ladies and Sisters under her superintendence, who were now deprived of her gentle and impartial government; by the medical officers, whom she had promptly obeyed and cordially assisted, and by the patients who regarded her (as they did us all) with affectionate respect. The day preceding her departure Lord William Paulet's *aide-de-camp* visited us, to express Lord William's sense of the valuable services rendered by her to the hospital in his command.

The day she left us was very stormy, so that she had great difficulty in reaching the steamer lying in the Golden Horn. All the patients in the convalescent hospital able to walk came down to the quay to cheer her off as she left, the medical and other officers were assembled to bid her goodbye, and with many a heartfelt good wish and fervent blessing she was speeded on her way.

When she was gone our next step was to prepare for the new party of ladies and nurses. Before Miss Stanley left, we had decided it was necessary to find new quarters, for two reasons: first, owing to the increased staff of medical and other officers there was not sufficient room in the hospital for their accommodation without the rooms we occupied; secondly, our health had suffered so severely from our quarters being in the hospital, that we felt to be outside its walls would be far more desirable.

The first house beyond the Riding School was examined and found to answer the purpose very well, except that the Turk who owned it objected to letting it even at the enormous rent he asked. It was necessary to apply through our embassy to the *Sultan*. Had we been French we should have gained possession in a few days, but British negotiations in the East are carried on with dignified slowness; so, during the week that followed Miss Stanley's departure we were kept in daily expectation of hearing that the house was in our possession, and were daily disappointed.

Two days after Miss Stanley left one of the two remaining paid nurses sickened with fever; her companion was required to nurse her, so that the whole work of both hospitals fell upon the one lady and the ten Sisters, one of whom was still dangerously ill. That lady can never forget the intense anxiety of that week, short as the time was. Every day precious lives hung in the balance; never can she forget the indefatigable manner in which the Sisters of Mercy carried on the work of the hospital. Already tasked beyond their strength, they willingly and cheerfully took the additional work which the departure, illness, and death among the lady staff had thrown on their hands, and so admirable was their method, so unremitting their skill, that no patient in the hospital (it may be confidently said) suffered from the diminution of numbers.

As the time for the arrival of the new party drew so near that they might be daily expected, and there was still no news from the embassy that we might have the house, matters looked serious. We had especially shrunk from bringing the new party fresh from sea air into rooms impregnated with fever. Of our four rooms, in one the nurse was lying ill of fever, in another Miss Smythe had died. However, there now appeared no choice.

By applying to Dr. Humphrey, P.M.O., we obtained the temporary use of a room at the end of the new and unoccupied ward, situated at the extreme end of the building; this we made a dormitory for some of the paid nurses under charge of a lady, the rest we prepared accommodation for in our three rooms, the fourth having our invalid and her nurse.

At the end of this week a large number of invalids went to England, which somewhat thinned the wards. It was always a great labour when the invalids went, as we had to give them articles of clothing from our free-gift store. Sometimes we had not enough to give. There was a great want of brushes and combs among the men. Soldiers are generally supposed to carry them in their knapsacks, but almost all the sick who passed through our hands in the winter and spring had lost their knapsacks either in the camp or on the passage down; they were therefore quite destitute. We applied to Mr. Stow, the *Times* Commissioner, for brushes and combs, and many other articles we required for the men. He sent them immediately.

Previous to this date Mr. Stow visited us, informed us he had taken Mr. Macdonald's place, and was ready to give us any help we required from the *Times* Fund. We gladly availed ourselves of the offer, and we can thankfully bear witness to numberless comforts and necessaries supplied by the *Times* Fund to the sick. Mr. Stow appeared a person admirably suited for his post. He visited the hospital constantly and thoroughly, gaining a complete insight into its working.

There were other visitors to the hospital, who paid their visits once a fortnight or so, attended by a long train of authorities, and though doubtless it was meant for the best, yet it seemed impossible for these to gain such a knowledge of the real wants of the hospitals as a man who came and went at any hour and without observation. Great was my astonishment upon being told one day by a distinguished person that the *Times* Commissioner was a "dangerous person." I made no answer to the remark.

Living as we then were amid scenes of sickness and death, tending the wasted forms of those whom want and neglect had brought to this dire extremity, seeing as we *hourly* did the flower of the British Army cut down in the prime of their youth and strength—as we saw those cherished in the heart of their country lacking daily the common comforts lavished on the sick of English hospitals—my heart was too sick and weary to enter into any controversy about the authorities and the *Times* Commissioner. I only knew one let the men die for want of things—the other provided them; the one *talked*, and the other *acted*.

I could not help thinking that I cared not where the things came from so that they did come somehow; so, I went straight to the "dangerous person," who was pacing up and down the barrack-yard, with an air as if he cared very little what people thought of him, and laid a list of our present wants before him.

"These things are promised," I said, "but we shall have to wait very long for them, even if we do get them at all." Mr. Stow wrote them down in his note-book; by that time the next day they were on the spot. This energy was one of Mr. Stow's characteristics. A thing once mentioned to him he never forgot, and never rested till it was done. He was particularly anxious on the subject of washing; it was a great evil, but at that time there was no remedy. Mr. Stow asked if we thought washing machines from England would be useful, but we told him there was no place to put them in, and then the plan would require much superintendence, for which we had no time to spare—we had not even time to search into the full extent of the abuse itself.

However, his attention having been once drawn to it, he never lost sight of it. As time went on, we used to laugh among ourselves, and say, "Here comes Mr. Stow, and now we shall have something about the washing." If Mr. Stow had lived to return to Constantinople he would have found Koulali much improved in that, as well as in all other respects.

The last visit Mr. Stow paid us was when the fruit was just coming into season, strawberries especially. We told him how the men longed for them, and he gave us leave to buy as many as we wanted. The new purveyor-in-chief being then in office, Mr. Stow seemed to feel his services were no longer wanted to the same extent. He said he knew Mr. Robertson would see that every requisite was furnished, and that matters would soon be on a different footing.

He went to the camp, and among the many who regretted the untimely death of one so talented were some at Koulali, who will ever remember his untiring exertions in his country's cause, his extreme courtesy, and the kind and friendly manner with which he cheered on the sinking hearts that had struggled through that time of misfortune.

CHAPTER 7

The Plague of Rats

April the 8th was Easter Sunday, but it, like joyous Christmas, fell strangely on us. On this day I sent Papafée, our interpreter, to Constantinople to be on the spot when the steamer was telegraphed by which we expected our staff of ladies and nurses, that he might go on board and bring two of the former to Koulali at once, in order that I might have an hour or two's warning to complete our preparations for the large party.

April 9th.—The morning passed away without Papafée's return, and I concluded the steamer had not come in; but at noon we were startled with the news that the admiral's small steamer, with "nurses onboard," was alongside. I ran down to the beach and welcomed the party to their strange home and untried work. My first inquiry was why Papafée had not obeyed orders and brought me timely news. He, with violent gesticulations, excused himself, declaring he was the first who boarded the *Osiris*, but shortly after he had done so there came a messenger from the embassy, desiring the lady in whose charge the party had travelled to come to Lady Stratford's immediately; this she did and stayed there to breakfast, and thus the delay had arisen.

The party had brought bedsteads and bedding with them from Marseilles, and this with the necessary number of boxes for so large a party was an appalling incursion into our crowded rooms. The corridor was already nearly full of presses, boxes, and some large cases of books, which could not be placed in the chaplain's quarters. There was no library, and the books were all carried to the chaplains, from whom we received them for distribution. The new party were twenty-five in number when they left England; five were left at Scutari, so that twenty joined our staff; they consisted of six ladies and fourteen hired nurses.

Before the new party could enter upon their respective work, it was necessary a lady superintendent, in the room of Miss Stanley, should be appointed. Up to this juncture the nurses in Koulali hospitals were nominally under Miss Nightingale's charge. She now resigned this charge, and we were informed of the fact by a letter to that effect from Mr. Bracebridge, and afterwards by a verbal communication from Lord William Paulet, who said that now the appointment of the Superintendent of Nurses would rest in his hands, and that she would be responsible only to him, except in the details of hospital work, in which she was under obedience to the principal medical officer.

Three days afterwards Miss Hutton, one of the ladies of the new party, was nominated as Lady Superintendent, by Lord William Paulet.

Before commencing their work Miss Hutton laid before Dr. Humphrey, the principal medical officer, the rules for our work in the hospital, which had been drawn up by Miss Stanley previous to her departure. They were the following:

1. The nurses in charge of the wards should take care that the orders of the medical officers concerning ventilation are carried out, that everything should be clean and in order, and they should see to the cleanliness of the patients' beds.

2. They should see that the diet and medicine ordered by the medical officers be given at the appointed times, and that all their directions be strictly attended to.

3. The nurses will be in the wards when the surgeons pay their morning visits, in order to receive any directions, they may give. They will be ready to wash or dress wounds, change poultices, apply fomentations, etc., as may be required.

4. The strictest attention is to be paid to the orders of the medical officers; nothing is to be given to the patients without their permission.

5. To each ward will be appointed a lady, a Sister of Mercy, and a nurse. The lady and nurse will enter and leave the ward together. They will visit the wards morning, afternoon, and evening, as they are wanted.

6. One lady will undertake the charge of the store-room, giving out whatever may be needed to the ladies, Sisters, and nurses for their wards. The same lady will also superintend the giving out of the extra diets for the patients.

7. Books shall not be given or lent to the patients by ladies or nurses unless received for that purpose from the chaplain of the communion to which the patient belongs.

The superintendent then assigned to each person her work, divided the wards between ladies and nuns, thereby releasing the overworked Sisters from the double charge they had been holding for some weeks. This week the only lady left of Miss Stanley's band sickened, apparently with fever, and the superintendent had her instantly removed to the new house (which had been at last obtained), but only one room of which was ready for occupancy. The lady very much benefited by this removal to a room where she could be quiet and alone. The relief could only be imagined by those who had passed many months as we had sleeping and living in large numbers in one room in sickness and in health. The change of air or other causes, by God's blessing, gave the illness a favourable turn, and she resumed her work in a fortnight.

Ere this the necessary repairs were completed, and the whole body of ladies and nurses (with the exception of the sick nurse, who had had a relapse, and could not move), left their two rooms in the hospital and took possession of the house. It was a very pretty and convenient one. We called it the "Home on the Bosphorus;" but as this was rather too long a title it always went by the name of the "Home." Some apartments in the right wing were occupied by Dr. and Mrs. Tice; two small rooms were allotted by Lady Stratford's express desire to the senior chaplain of the Church of England. The apartments occupied by Dr. Tice and the chaplain adjoined our dining-room, but were otherwise divided from the rest of the house.

The house was built according to Turkish fashion, corridors on every floor, with rooms opening out of them; the kitchen separate from the house, adjoining it the bathhouse. This was out of repair, and it would have taken too much time and expense to have put it to rights. The front rooms quite overhung the Bosphorus. We could see the water through the chinks of the rafters in the front part of the room.

In a violent storm which occurred about this time, when the quiet Bosphorus lashed itself into fury, and when no *caique* would venture out, our rooms rocked as if they were cabins on board ship, and the new party were quite alarmed, and declared they expected to be in the Bosphorus soon; those who knew the climate assured them this was mild to winter storms at Therapia. Another earthquake occurred about this time, but it was not so alarming as the first.

From the first our house shared the fate of other Turkish houses—it was overrun with rats. They galloped about the ceiling with a sound as of a regiment of horse. When we opened the cupboards, we saw them disappearing into their holes. The devastation they wrought in the store-room was terrible; every morning beheld the lady who acted as housekeeper mourning over her losses and with no prospect of redress. At night they walked about our bedrooms, jumped upon our pillows, and quite broke the stillness of night. They would jump from stair to stair, sounding like a heavy man's footstep; they appeared to hammer and drive in nails, and saw and hack, till we could hardly believe they were only rats.

Often did we rise, thinking there must be human beings moving about, but found it was only our usual visitors. One night a lady left a biscuit in the pocket of her dress, in the morning the dress was eaten through and the biscuit gone. At length we heard rat-traps were in the stores. We eagerly asked for some. The first night they were used three were caught in one room, and from this time the store-room was better guarded, as we put the trap on the hole and every night a rat came and was killed. But nothing was able really to subdue the numbers, and there is not a Turkish house which is not overrun with them. Those we caught were like English rats.

We will now give an account of the routine of our life. When May opened the sickness and deaths had considerably abated, and our system had become more organised and our hours regular. It should here be mentioned that on April the 21st three ladies and seven nurses joined us. Our numbers were therefore twenty-three nurses, (including the sick one), ten ladies, and ten Sisters of Mercy. The Sisters, as before mentioned, lived in rooms at the General Hospital.

At the ladies' Home we assembled at eight o'clock for prayers, read by our superintendent, then followed breakfast. At nine the bell for work rang. We all assembled; each lady called the nurse under her charge to accompany her to her ward, or kitchen, or linen stores (we never allowed the nurses to go out alone, unless with special permission); and in five minutes all the different groups were on their way to the hospital. At two the ladies and their nurses returned home, unless there were cases who could not safely be left to the orderlies' charge to watch them, and then the lady, or Sister, in whose ward the case was, either stayed herself or appointed a nurse whom she could trust; but, generally speaking, we thought it better on all accounts to be absent from the wards for an hour or two.

At half-past two we dined, the ladies in one room, the nurses in another, with a lady at the head of their table. The ladies took it by turns, a week about, to superintend all the meals of the nurses. At half-past four the bell summoned us to return to the hospital. Some went sooner than this to the kitchen and linen store.

At seven we returned to tea; then one lady—we took it in turns—went out with the nurses for a walk; now and then, for a treat, in *caiques*, to the sweet waters, or Bebec. At nine the chaplain of the Church of England came and read part of the evening service. Those who wished for it took some supper ere they went to their rooms. Of course, such events as the arrival of sick, or extreme sickness in the hospital, would sometimes break the routine. So passed our lives for weeks and months.

We found our walks to and from the hospital rather inconvenient in the wet, and also the extreme heat, for it was on the banks of the

Bosphorus that we had to walk under a burning sun. Umbrellas were at a premium, for those bought in Pera were made so slightly they were continually breaking, and then we had to wait till someone went across to buy some more. Those who possessed such treasures as English umbrellas treasured them with great care, but we had great reason to be thankful for the good health that we all enjoyed. We had only one case of serious illness among either ladies or nurses.

Exposed as we were to contagious diseases, we greatly attribute this, under God's blessing, to our living outside the hospital walls, and also to the frequent exercise we took. It was often very fatiguing, after a long day in the wards, to escort the long train of nurses for an evening walk. They were rather exigent in their wishes as to where they should go. Some wished to climb the hills to catch the breeze, while others declared they could only walk along the shore, while the oldest of the party (and rather a character amongst us) had yearnings after a *krogue* as she termed a *caique*.

A favourite walk with all was, however, to a neighbouring village called ("Greek town." It used to amuse the nurses extremely to see the manners and customs of the inhabitants. On one occasion we found them all keeping festival; it was one of their numerous fete days, and apparently the day's celebration had something to do with a well possessing some medicinal qualities.

Not far from this was a pretty garden, where were assembled some Greek peasantry in their gayest costumes listening to music and merrily conversing with each other. The only remarkable feature in the dress of the Greek women is their head-dress, which is profusely ornamented with flowers, lace, and ribbon, a short gauze veil thrown over it. This is only among the peasantry. The Greek ladies are rapidly adopting Parisian style.

One day, shortly after we had got into regular work, our interpreter came running in and said, "Make haste, and you will see a sight which no English ladies have ever seen before!" Those of our party who happened to be at home followed him, and he took us into the next house, a few yards from our own. In the courtyard we found a large assemblage of Greeks and Turks, who all smiled and seemed very much pleased at our appearance, and conducted us into the house and into a large room on the ground floor.

What a picture it was! On the cushioned divan, which ran along one side of the room, sat three venerable-looking *imaums*, in flowing robes, long beards, white turbans, and with *chibouque*. On their right and left, upon the divan, were seated a dozen boys, of ages varying from six to twelve, whose dress marked them of high rank. In a conspicuous position among these was a tiny boy, about four years old. He wore a little coat of crimson velvet, embroidered in gold; trousers and vest to match; a leather band, richly worked, round his waist, from which hung a tiny sword. On his head a velvet *fez*, beautifully embroidered, with a heavy gold tassel, completed his attire.

On a small desk before the *imaums* were several large books in the Turkish language. One was lying open. Below the divan were rows of little Turks, all dressed alike in the coat and trousers and crimson cloth *fez*. They sat in rows on the floor like an English infant-school, and their little red caps made them look at a distance like a bed of poppies. Truth to say, they behaved a great deal better than the same number of little Britons would have done. Our entrance attracted their attention. Only for an instant they gave us a look, then settled themselves again. And now one *imaum* called up one boy after another to read a sentence out of the great book; when he had finished his sentence all the school cried out, "*Amen*."

At length the little boy whose dress we have described descended from his seat and stood at the *imaum's* feet, then slowly repeated each word after the *imaums*. He accomplished a sentence, a very loud "*Amen!*" followed, and there was a buzz and a smile on everyone's face as if some feat had been accomplished. The child returned to his place and the other boys went up in turns for their lesson.

How we were beckoned out of the room. Outside we found two pretty Greek girls, who by smiles and signs invited us upstairs to the *haréem*. We accepted the invitation, and soon arrived at the upper corridor of the house, from which numerous rooms opened. Here we were received by a number of Turkish ladies, children, and slaves, one or two other Greeks, as well as our conductress. Here we for the first time saw the Turkish women without their *feridgees* or *yashmacs*.

There was no furniture of any kind in the rooms but divans; the floors were matted and everything looked beautifully clean. We were seated on the divan and the ladies looked well at us, and inspected the textures of our dresses. They treated us with the greatest courtesy, and seemed delighted at the visit. Soon they brought us pipes and began to smoke themselves, and evidently watched to see what we should do.

We accordingly made an effort at smoking, but thought it unnecessary to do more than smoke for a minute or two for politeness' sake, and when we laid down the pipes a general burst of laughter showed their amusement. Then came coffee, in tiny silver cups, and after this we rose to take our leave. But, no, we could not go. A small table and chairs were now brought in, and some Turkish sweetmeats and pastry offered. We were obliged to taste, or it would have been an affront.

After this we again prepared to take our leave. A great deal of talking went on between the Turkish and Greek women. The result was that when we reached the courtyard, where our interpreter waited for us, the Greek girls told him that the Turkish ladies hoped we would honour them again that evening and bring all the others with us. We said we were too large a party, but this made them miserable—so the superintendent consented.

At seven in the evening, they sent in to know if we were not coming. At that hour a large number of the party were disengaged from work, and these went in. We were received with great delight; chairs were placed in the corridors, and they seemed hardly to know how to make enough of us. There were a large number of Turkish women now and many Greeks. There were several of the former strikingly beautiful, but a great number of the others had a sickly look, and evidently their beauty soon faded. Now they brought two large brass candlesticks, six feet high, with candles to match, and placed them in the centre of the room. We sat round by the wall on our chairs—the Turkish ladies in groups on the floor.

On the floor, opposite the lights, were three slaves with tambourines, who now began a hideous kind of music; the dancing girls entered and began to dance round the candlesticks. They danced very gracefully, but after a short time it grew very monotonous, although the interest the Turkish women took seemed not to flag for a minute. When this was ended, they had some game among themselves, in which a key formed a principal part. We could not make out what it was, further than it was some joke about the key of the *haréem*.

At the conclusion of this game, some of the ladies approached us and made signs that they knew we were doctors, and they were very ill and wanted advice— they believed all English were doctors. Of course, we made the most of our medical knowledge; sent for our little medicine chest, and prescribed some simple medicines, which could do no harm and which, with so much faith, might prove as efficacious as Parr's Life Pills or other wonders in England. After this ceremony we took our departure.

This festival was on the occasion of the son and heir of the house going to school for the first time; the father of the child being dead, the little boy was a person of great importance. We should mention that he was brought into the *haréem* and made a great pet of, and much admired. He was a pretty, intelligent-looking little fellow. The dress of many of the ladies was very handsome; silk, or gauze, with a great deal of embroidery and many jewels: the hair also much dressed, with gauze, artificial flowers, &c. Gloves evidently were considered the height of fashion among the ladies. They were only worn by ladies of high rank, who considered them a great ornament, and always liked them of bright colours.

CHAPTER 8

The Old Age of Sickness

We will now lead our readers through the wards, and endeavour to describe their arrangement and the order of their work. Ward No. 1 was called the "detachment ward," this meaning that which was occupied by the body of men stationed at the hospital. No. 2 was empty, the surgical patients having been removed from it till the horses could be dislodged from the stables beneath, which had rendered this ward very unhealthy. No. 3 was the fever ward; both upper and lower corridors had been filled with British sick for some time, the Russian prisoners (with the exception of two bad cases left in the surgical ward) having been removed towards the end of March to the arsenal at Constantinople.

No. 3 ward lower was under charge of a lady and nurse; No. 3 upper under charge of a Sister and nurse. The floor of No. 3 lower ward was brick, a large stove stood in the middle, and one table, which was of course not sufficient for the wants of the long ward. On each side of the ward, under the gallery, a wooden boarding was laid; on this were the trestle beds. The heads of these beds were open bars, on the top of which was a narrow ledge which held their medicine bottles, their drinking cup and dish (these two latter articles at least ought to have been there, but there was a sad deficiency in them).

Over the bed was nailed a printed card, the blank spaces of which were filled up with writing; the information given on it was as follows: Name, regiment, date of admission, age, disease, religion—the last was inserted respectively, Church of England, Roman Catholic, Presbyterian. The benefit of this latter regulation was much felt in the hospital by the chaplains, ladies, and Sisters, as they could thus each gain the knowledge of those belonging to their own faith without questioning the patients.

The card over their bed was not originally intended to bear this record of their faith, but the regulation was early made on account of the mistakes and almost absurdities which the want of it sometimes caused. There were few things so painful to us as the constantly being obliged to ask this question before we dared lend a book or speak a word of religious consolation to our patients, and it did them no good—sometimes causing a smile, and sometimes a look of annoyance, on their faces.

"I'm sick to death of that question," said a poor fellow very wearily one day to a lady; he did not the least intend it as rudeness, but the sergeant of the ward unfortunately took into his head that it was so, and after the lady had left, he thought it necessary to report to the medical officer that this patient had spoken rudely to one of the ladies. The physician was much displeased of course, and immediately as a punishment knocked off his "extras," *i.e.*, reduced him to his original diet of bread and tea. The next day, in going my rounds, the poor man called me to his bedside and burst into tears, asking me if I could tell him where Miss ——— lived, as he wanted to ask her to come and speak to him.

I replied that she lived in the same room as myself, and I would tell her to come; when she did so, he again burst into tears, and humbly apologised for his unintentional rudeness, saying, "It's not the extras I care for m'am, but having been thought to speak rudely to one of you kind ladies." She quite reassured him when she replied that the sergeant had been entirely mistaken, and that she never for a moment thought such a thing.

At one end of the ward was a long dresser, on which plates and tins, knives and forks, were kept; this dresser possessed cupboards in the lockers, two of which were assigned to the ladies' or Sisters' use, to keep linen or wine and other articles likely to be needed in a hurry. The daily routine of the work was for the Sister and lady to go round their wards with their surgeon and receive his direction, then give out the wine; it came in a large pail. Port wine was much used, one and two gills, respectively, being measured out; the extras were distributed. The regular dinner hour was half-past twelve, breakfast at seven, tea at four, but of course serious cases had to be attended to at all times, and food given to them constantly in small quantities.

The work was laborious no doubt, but now the agony of distress had passed away. Spring had come at last, and the woe of that terrible winter was already becoming like a dream. The party of ladies and nurses who arrived on April 9th saw scarcely anything of that sad distress, at least at Koulali. I am not acquainted whether the change at Scutari took place at the same time, though my impression is that it did; certainly, with us at Easter the tide of death and disease suddenly turned after we sent home invalids in Holy week. We were never again overcrowded; mortality began visibly to decrease.

The unremitting exertions of the medical officer to conquer the diseases by skilful treatment, better food, and constant nursing, were blessed; and those who had passed through those dreary months felt as if they indeed heard the words, "It is enough, stay now thy hand." No one can imagine but they who experienced it the oppressive hopeless feeling the sight of that great mortality had brought, I suppose similar to that felt by those who have been spectators of the destruction wrought by the plague in foreign countries, and the cholera in our own.

To return to our subject; this emergency passed away, and our life was a regular routine of work and rest (except on occasions of extraordinary pressure) following each other in order; but whether in the strain of overwork or the steady fulfilment of our arduous duty, there was one bright ray ever shed over it, one thing that made labour light and sweet, and this was the respect, affection, and gratitude of the men. No words can tell it rightly, for it was unbounded, and as long as we stayed among them it never changed.

Familiar as our presence became to them, though we were in and out of the wards day and night they never forgot the respect due to our sex and position. Standing by those in bitter agony, when the force of old habits is great, or by those in the glow of returning health, or walking up the wards among orderlies and sergeants, never did a word which could offend a woman's ear fall upon ours. Even in the barrack-yard, passing by the guard-room or entrances, where stood groups of soldiers smoking and idling, the moment we approached all coarseness was hushed; and this lasted, not a week or a month, but the whole of my twelvemonth's residence, and my experience is also that of all my companions.

With some brilliant exceptions the manner in which the war has been conducted is a source of humiliation to England; but yet she has something left to boast of in her noble sons—brave before their enemies, gentle to their countrywomen—yes, many a time have our hearts bounded with joyful pride in our countrymen. Many instances of their nobility of character might be given; we select the most remarkable as we pass through each ward.

In No. 3 lower was M———; he was the only one seriously ill in the ward, so that a lady sat up one night for his sake only this he knew, and he was quite distressed about it, and did nothing but cry, for he was very weak. "Really, M———," said she, it is useless for me to sit up if you are going to make yourself ill about it in this foolish way. I am quite strong enough to sit up till the morning, when I shall go to bed; but it is mere waste of time to come if you are going to cry in this way all night."

"I can't abeer it," said he, "to see you running about and tiring yourself for me." At length she succeeded in quieting him, and when the morning came, finding him better, she left him.

Shortly after the lady of the ward came in to her daily work, when he eagerly enquired after his night nurse; and though he was assured of her perfect health and well-being, again did his tears begin to flow at the remembrance of what he had taken into his head to fancy was such very hard work. He was an orphan, and on his return to England had no home but the workhouse; his constitution being shattered, we fear for ever. Perhaps it was his lonely lot in this world that made him cling to us, and seem so astonished at any one caring for his comfort.

It was the look of surprise on his face when he first came down from the Crimea at the least little act of kindness that affected one more than anything; he had evidently not been much accustomed to receive it through life, but he always said, with a smile on his face, that it was "all right—God knew best." In this ward was Walter, a little drummer boy about twelve; he was a pretty child, with a remarkably clear sweet voice, and had been admitted into the singing class; he was very much spoiled by the soldiers, and had grown saucy and conceited. He caught fever, and came into No. 3 lower. When he was getting better, he said to the lady:

"I have been a very naughty boy before I was ill, but I mean to change now. I promised father, when I came away, that I would read the Bible every day, and say my prayers, and I have kept my promise in a sort of way, for I always did it; but then I chose out the very shortest chapters, and said my prayers as fast as I could, just to get over it somehow, but I shan't do that again if I get well."

Afterwards he used to bring the lady beautiful flowers, as a childish mark of affection and gratitude for her having nursed him.

Another patient in this ward had a broken jaw, which had been struck by a heavy blow at the taking of the Redan, and, in consequence, though he recovered his health, he could not eat the usual hospital diet, and was entirely dieted from the ladies' kitchen with rice pudding, beef tea, arrowroot, &c. He was very anxious to be sent to England, but one day he said to the lady of his ward, in a melancholy tone,

"I shall never get sent home if you are so kind to me, and feed me up like this, for my arms has grown so fat; and when the chief doctors come their rounds to examine the men for England, they takes hold of them and feels them, and then they don't think I'm bad enough to be 'invalided home.'"

"Well," said the lady, laughing, "I suppose I had better leave off taking care of you!"

He did not seem at all certain whether it would not be better to starve a little, for the sake of getting home. However, at last his wish was granted, and he was invalided home. He told the lady, the night before he set sail for home, that his widowed mother in England would pray for her.

The surgeons were of course anxious to keep the men in the East as long as there was the least hope of their recovery; but it used to be weary work to be kept waiting month after month, with their constitutions so broken and shattered, that, in spite of all that was done for them, both by doctors and nurses, they were obliged to be dismissed home at last. The thought of going home seemed to pour new life into them for the time. Many of them used to come from the Crimea looking so worn and so *old*, it used to startle us sometimes when we glanced at the card above their head to see their real age. "You only twenty?"

"Yes, that's all," was the answer, "but we had a hard time of it up there!"

Our orderlies were a great help to us; they were always most respectful and obedient, though of course they needed constantly looking after. One of our nurses mistook their names, and always called them "Aldernies."

"Now, Alderney, run and get this beef tea warmed!"

"If you please, nurse, there's no fire, and the charcoal is all gone, and the Greeks 'as run over the brasier in the barrack-yard with their carts and 'as knocked off two of its legs!"

"Never mind that, Alderney, you can get a requisition for charcoal, and you can put up the brasier with stones, and get the water hot. If we want a fire we must have a fire, so that's the long and short of it!"

One day a man was brought in to No. 3 lower from the guard-room, where he had been confined for the night, in consequence of having been found drunk on duty. On being put into the guard-room those who had charge of the prisoners were so struck by the strangeness of his manner that they thought best to watch him; and fortunately, they did so, for he had loaded his musket and intended to destroy himself. It was a sad case of *delirium tremens*—he never recovered his senses while with us. He more than once rushed out of the ward, managed to elude the sentries at the entrance, and attempted to throw himself into the Bosphorus, but our orderlies followed and brought him back.

When in the ward he was very quiet, seldom spoke, except to tell the lady that he was pursued by evil spirits, and had sinned beyond the hope of forgiveness; in vain she tried to cheer and comfort him. The chaplain, too, did all in his power, and some of the patients were very kind—trying to amuse and draw him out of himself, and to persuade him to walk with them in the barrack yard. He promised one of the lads that he would go with him to church, but when he got to the door he rushed back again, saying someone was going to kill him.

Poor fellow, it was terrible to witness his remorse, and listen to his bitter self-accusations. We vainly assured him of the pardon and peace which he seemed to have lost the power of believing. Sometimes he would repeat the Lord's prayer after the lady, and listen to a hymn, and say it was very nice; but he soon relapsed into his former despondency, and the doctors, after trying all they could to restore him to health, were finally obliged to send him to England under careful charge, lest he should drown himself, as I fear he intended.

In No. 3 lower was also another very interesting case—a young lad, with whose quiet and really gentlemanly manners we were much struck. He seemed much superior to those around him, but was so reserved that he rarely spoke, though he appeared unhappy, and as if he needed sympathy. At last, he confided to us his history. He was the son of an English gentleman; had been sent to school at Rugby.

In a wayward moment he had enlisted and had left England without the knowledge of his father or his friends. After a little persuasion the chaplain prevailed upon him to write and tell his father the truth, and we had the satisfaction of knowing before he left the hospital that he had obtained his father's forgiveness. We believe he eventually went up to Sebastopol.

Another case was a young man with very bad typhus fever. He was not expected to recover. His mind continually wandered, but he was very obedient and docile. He used often to sing hymns, such, we would fancy, as he had learned in his childhood at some village church in England, for he was evidently a country lad. He was extremely fond of repeating over and over again to the lady and the orderlies that God was very good, very good indeed, and that he loved Him.

He found great relief from having large lumps of ice applied to his head; he was very grateful, telling the lady that she was like a mother to him, and better than a mother, for what he knew. Much to her surprise he recovered, and slowly regained his strength. He was so childlike in his obedience and affection, that she felt quite sorry, for her own sake, to see him quit her ward for the convalescent hospital.

Another poor fellow came down from the Crimea, after some months spent in the hospital there, looking utterly shattered and worn out, and apparently about fifty or thereabouts, but on looking at his card we found he was only twenty. He rallied for a few days, but sank at last. The day he died he told the lady of his ward that he had a little money which he wished to leave to some friend of his in Ireland, who had been the same to him as a father. He had no near relations living. The lady asked the *commandant* about it, who said that unless he made a will his money would of course go to the next of kin.

The soldiers have now a little book provided for each of them by the quartermaster, in which they set down their accounts, &c., and in which are written several military regulations. At the end there is a form for making a will. The corporal of the ward wrote out, according to the *commandant's* order, a copy of this, and then the poor fellow was required to sign his name in the presence of the medical officer.

But, alas! his mind was now wandering, and the death dew was standing on his forehead. He just rallied sufficiently, however, a short time after, to sign his name. It was so touching to see the eager way in which the trembling hand fulfilled its task. True, it was but a pound or so he had to leave, but he seemed so anxious to show this last little testimony of affection and gratitude to one who had loved him and had been kind to the orphan boy when father and mother were laid in the grave.

In the intervals of reason that last day he got the lady to write a letter for him to this friend, but she was obliged to finish it after his death; one sentence he bade her write was, "I have gone through a power of hardships up at the front." His worn face did indeed speak of a power of hardships.

He was a Roman Catholic, and the lady therefore requested the Sister of Mercy in the gallery above to come down and pray by him, which she very often did during his illness; he died very peacefully, while she was reading the last prayers by his bedside, and without a groan.

Another man was quite an example to his regiment for his good conduct and sobriety, he had attained the rank of corporal. He had a very pleasant manner of talking to his fellow comrades, and persuading them not to indulge in drink. He had been a long time in the service, and, his health being shattered, was very anxious to return home to his wife and child: but he always said, smiling, that he was ready to stay if necessary: that he knew for certain all would be right, whichever way it was.

He told us so quaintly one day that it was "all through drink he came to be a good man." It sounded a strange anomaly, and we almost smiled, but the explanation followed. He had some years back, when a very young man, got into trouble through this habit; good advice was offered him. The captain of his regiment established a school, where those who wished to escape the temptation to drink which idleness offers, might find instruction and employment. He entered the school, broke through his bad habit, and said "he blessed God for the day he began to do so."

After his return to England he wrote the following letter to the lady of his ward:—

Dear Madam.—With gratitude to Almighty God I arrived in dear old England once again, after a passage of fourteen days; beautiful weather the whole way; good accommodation on board the *Niagara* for the sick and wounded. My pains are very troublesome at times. I am afraid I am worn out as far as military duties are concerned. It will be a great disadvantage to me to be discharged at the present time, but if it is so ordered I am satisfied with my lot. I feel it my duty as a Christian to submit to the Divine Providence of God, for I can truly say I have been brought by a way that I knew not, and by that same good Providence I am restored to my dear wife and family.

I return you a thousand thanks for your kind care over me in my affliction. The Lord will reward you, because He has promised so to do. He seems to raise up friends for me in all parts.

Please to tell Miss —— that I can never forget her kindness in giving me the advice and the address of her relatives. How many happy times have I spent in Koulali Hospital Church! the daily morning service was a blessing to me, and at the table of the Lord He was always present with me.

You will please tell the Rev. Mr. Coney that I return him my thanks for his spiritual care over my soul there, and that I trust he will have many souls given him for his care and labour, although discouragement is around him.

The joy and happiness of meeting my friends once more makes me almost forget what trials and hardships I went through. I am thankful my life is spared. I am content with my lot, but I am so much shook that I am happy to say I shall not be sent out again. I am at present attending hospital; I go for medicine three times a day. If the weather was not so wet it might be better for me; still, I must not dictate to the Almighty what weather we are to have.

And now, dear madam, you will excuse me if I have in any way transgressed in freedom in writing; my prayers shall ever be offered up for you, and all who belong to you, and you are a treasure to your family and the British Army in the East.

I remain your humble servant,

———— ————

2nd Battalion Rifle Brigade, Aldershott Camp.

Chapter 9

Russian Prisoners

The extreme youth of some of our patients and their childishness was a great amusement to the orderlies, especially the Irish ones, who delighted in having, what they called, a spree with some of them.

"Now, Dick, my boy, what would you like this morning—a bit of plum-pudding or a few sugar-plums? Ask the lady for some, she's sure to get them for you if you ask her."

"I'll tell you what, my boy, you better had stayed at home along with your mother than come a knocking out in this country; a bit of a chap like you ain't fit for such rough work."

One of the No. 3 orderlies was quite a character, and his eccentricities were a great amusement to us; his name was Rooke. Part of his business was to fetch the extras from the ladies' store-room for his ward; when he came back with a pail full of something in each hand, and his shirt-front remarkably enlarged from the bottles of soda-water he had ingeniously filled it with; he used to look of great importance, making as much noise as he could in setting them down, and calling out to the nurse—

"How, miss, here they be, and I hopes you 'as got enough today."

Whenever he had forgotten anything, he had a peculiar way of rubbing his head and pulling his hair and trying to make excuses. He was a capital nurse, and full of rough kindness to the patients. He was generally so merry and full of Irish fun that it was a surprise to see him one morning looking sad and unhappy; but on inquiry we found that he had just received a letter telling him of the death of his wife, and asking what was to be done with his three little children.

He still went on doing his hospital work as attentively as before, but evidently with an aching heart. He said that he had known his poor wife ever since she was a little girl, that his mother and hers had lived in two adjoining cottages, and that they had been brought up and played together as children, and now she had died far away from him after a short illness. He used to save his money to send home to her and the children, looking forward with such hope to seeing them all again, and now he seemed utterly cast down, and the joking with his patients was at an end for some time.

At length, however, he somewhat recovered his spirits. In spite of his many good qualities he was remarkable for being as dirty and untidy in his dress as he dared without quite outraging military discipline.

One day General Storks and Mr. Stafford were coming round the hospital—everybody was astir—I think it was the general's first public inspection after he succeeded Lord William Paulet in command: such a clearing of wards and such a brushing up of everything took place. The lady at the extras store-room was serving out requisitions as usual when Rooke was the first on the spot to get his, and to her astonishment he was dressed up and in full regimentals. The expected visit had slipped her memory, seeing it made no difference to her work.

"Why, Rooke, what is the matter?" said she.

"They've a dressed me up to see that big man as is coming, if you please, miss."

Presently Rooke walked into his ward with a pailful of lemonade, and, setting it down by the lady, said—

"There, miss, now we'll give him a drink: when he comes."

No sooner had the general's party left the hospital when Rooke the smart soldier returned, with evident satisfaction, to Rooke the untidy orderly.

No. 3 upper ward was under charge of Sister M—— O——, and also contained fever patients. It was a long gallery with tables and cupboards at the end. The corporal, who was ward-master, was idle and inefficient, and did not look after his orderlies, who of course became a riotous set. At one time the ward was dirty and neglected. Upon one occasion the ward-master insisted upon giving out the wine himself, instead of the lady; this was of course against rules altogether. The lady spoke to Dr. Beatson, who was staff-surgeon of the division. He instantly came in and told the ward-master to mind what he was about; if he disobeyed orders a second time he should go to the guard-room.

The superintendent, seeing the ward was one requiring peculiar care from the lady in charge, appointed Sister M—— A——, thinking this Sister the best nurse in the Barrack Hospital.

In a few weeks the whole aspect of No. 3 upper was changed— it was clean and in order. The Sister gained her usual influence over the orderlies—they loved and respected her so they would do anything to please her. In time she had a better ward-master.

It was astonishing the influence gained by the ladies and Sisters over the orderlies. Without their superintendence they were an idle, useless set of men, callous to the sufferings of those around them, not trying to learn their business, which was of course new to them, and regardless of carrying out the doctor's orders when they could do so without getting into disgrace; but under the Sisters' and ladies' hands they became an excellent set of nurses, forming that class of men-nurses of course essential in a military hospital.

A great drawback to this was, however, that often when one had a good orderly willing to learn, and had trained him into the way of waiting on the sick, he would be sent for to his regiment, his place supplied by another quite unused to hospital work, and with whom the teaching had to begin all over again.

One day a poor fellow was brought into No. 3 upper from a ship proceeding to Balaclava. He was an Italian, and could not speak a word either of French or English, and, although the surgeon of his ward could speak Italian, we could gather little of his history from his few dying words; for he was in the last stage of fever when brought into the hospital, and it was soon all over. He seemed so grateful for all that was done for him, and was so delighted to get a drink of lemonade, making signs to have plenty of sugar put in.

Another case up in this ward was a poor little sailor, who was also brought in from a ship going to Balaclava. He remained for a long time, and was eventually obliged to be sent to England with the military invalids. He was such a curious little man, very meek and quiet, but as frightened and nervous as a woman, always thinking himself much worse than he was in reality, speaking invariably in a tone of deep despondency, much to the vexation of the orderly who was especially directed to look after him night and day, and who was a great tall fellow, not apparently much afraid of anything or anybody.

He was most kind and attentive to the small sailor, but evidently much chagrined at his want of hope and courage; he also seemed to think it must be very discouraging to the Sister who attended to him, so whenever he saw her going up to the sailor he followed her and exhorted him very energetically to "spake up to the lady; don't be so down-hearted, man; spake up, man, spake up, she don't hear what you are a saying of; why don't ye cheer up a bit? ye'll never get well that rate; ye'll make yourself a deal worser being so low-spirited."

This was of course quite true, but the poor sailor did not seem much inclined, or indeed well able, to follow the advice of his soldier friend, though at last we did sometimes succeed in making him smile by declaring we would ask the commanding officer to make a soldier of him, and inquiring which regiment he would like to be enlisted in, picturing to him how brave he would look marching about with the coloured ribbons in his hat.

Writing their letters home for them was most amusing; very often they had not a word to say, but trusted entirely to the lady. "What shall I say?" we began with.

"Just anything at all you like, miss—just the same as you writes your own letters home. You knows how to make up a letter better than I do!"

"But how shall I begin?"

"My dear Thomas," the lady writes on, hoping dear Thomas is well, and informing him of the illness and whereabouts of his friend.

Then she inquires what relation the said "dear Thomas" is to him.

"Oh, he's just my father, miss!"

She suggests the propriety of addressing him by his usual title.

"Oh, never mind, miss; it's all the same—it will do very well!"

One of the men received a letter from his wife, entreating him in the most broken-hearted words, to allow her to come out and nurse him—that she was utterly miserable, could not sleep at night thinking of what he was enduring, and so on. The poor man very likely felt more than he cared to express, but he chose to treat it with apparent indifference, and almost amusement.

"That's just the way women talks—they're always a-wanting to do impossibilities. They fancies they can do anything! Oh, yes, they fancies it fast enough, but then, you see, they can't, so what's the good of it? I should like to see her come out here indeed! A pretty place for a woman by herself, and I shouldn't be able to see after her. She's much better at home, and I'll write and tell her once for all that it's impossible and no good whatever talking about it no more!"

Fortunately for the poor wife's feelings, his arm was too stiff to write that day, as he evidently intended to send her a severe reproof for her folly, rather forgetting in his wisdom the deep affection and anxiety contained in her earnest pleading to come and nurse him. As the post went out next day, he rather reluctantly accepted the Sister's proposal to write in his stead, and she, of course, took care to soften the refusal as much as possible, and poor Mrs. —— was very likely rather surprised at the unusually affectionate letter she received from her husband by that mail; and we must hope it in some little measure compensated for her disappointment, though, doubtless, a few stern lines merely granting her request would have been far preferable.

Many of our patients could not read a word, and were delighted when we had time to teach them, or to read a few verses to those who were too weak to hold a book or read long for themselves. They were grateful, too, for slates to write and sum upon; but talking of home and bygone days, and then of their warlike adventures in the Crimea, was their chief delight.

Lower Stable Ward was the first of the stables turned into a ward. When Turkish stables, they looked as if it would be impossible to convert them into habitations for Christians, but when Dr. Tice was Principal Medical Officer, he designed the improvement of this, and the execution reflected great credit on him: it became the best ward in the hospital, holding one hundred and fifty beds. It was large and airy, and had the unusual merit of being in the noonday heat of a Turkish summer perfectly cool.

The surgical cases were moved into it, and Dr. Temple was the officer in charge. This ward was entirely on the ground-floor, and very much wider than the other wards; therefore, though no division was made in the building, the superintendent divided the nursing between a lady and a Sister of Mercy, with nurses; the upper part of the ward, with its four rows of beds, was under Miss ——, and the lower under Sister M—— E——.

Under these ladies was one of the nurses who was a member of the Evangelical Alliance. She was an elderly person and very eccentric, but a very good nurse and a respectable woman, and gave great satisfaction to the Sister and lady under whom she worked.

Sister M ——E—— always spoke in high terms of her usefulness and diligence, and she in her turn expressed the most unbounded respect and affection for the Sister, whom she called an "angel upon earth."

In Sister M——E——'s division was a very interesting case—a Scotch Presbyterian of the name of Fisher. He came in to be treated with frost-bite, but the seeds of consumption were sown, and when the frostbite healed, he was evidently in a hopeless state. Never was the deceitful disease more plainly displayed than in that case. He lingered on month after month; now better, now apparently at the point of death; then the flame of life would suddenly spring up again, and a feverish strength made him imagine he was getting better. He wore away till his bones seemed ready to come through the skin. He was generally hungry and very fanciful.

There is something so affecting in watching by one whom one knows to be hovering on the verge of the grave, that everyone united in doing their best to alleviate the sufferings of his last hours on earth. Dr. Temple stayed long by his bedside endeavouring to find something to ease him. Fisher insisted that no medicines did him good save those made by Dr. Temple's own hands, and the kind surgeon always humoured him, and when his rounds were over went regularly to the dispensary to make up Fisher's medicines, and he used to invent a sort of effervescent draught, which was to be sweet as well, and was Fisher's great delight.

By Fisher's bedside even the rough orderlies grew gentle; one in particular was a great favourite with the poor sufferer, and Fisher was never happy when "Joe" was away. Dr. Temple told us we might give him anything he fancied; nothing could do him harm. Oatmeal porridge he used to long for very often, and Sister M—— E—— used to make it strictly according to his own directions, for he was very fanciful. He was always longing for something or other, and as far as our means allowed, he was supplied. Sister M—— E—— was most unremitting in her care of him, and the attention he required was constant.

Fisher was a singularly rough, quaint man, not given to many words of gratitude, but it was pleasing to see the way in which his pale wan face lit up when Sister M—— E—— made her appearance. His eyes followed her about the ward as she went to her other patients, and though he did not *say* much to express his sense of her services, yet a few words from him spoke a volume of the deep feeling that was in his breast. At last death came for him, he passed away without a visible pang, just worn out.

In the same division of the ward was Hickey, another most interesting case. He suffered from the same disease as Fisher, but its progress was far more rapid. Hickey was an Irish Catholic. His great longing was to go home; he was haunted by a perpetual fever to see his own green land once more, and when the deceitful rallyings of his complaint came his eye glittered as he talked of how soon he would be amongst his dear friends in the "old country;" and we who watched beside him saw in the very glitter of the eyes and flush on the pale cheek the signs that he no longer needed an earthly home. The goings to and fro of this world were soon to end for him.

To satisfy him, however, his name was put down in the list of "invalided home," but ere the time for the departure of the band came the fever strength was gone, and the death-struggle was at hand. The disappointment was sore, but he bore it meekly: neither that nor his severe struggles elicited a murmuring word. He was a deeply religious man, and attended to the duties of his religion with fervour, and though the love of life was strong within him he was "content to die," he said, "as it was God's holy will," and when death stood beside him he passed as a child falls asleep and on his pale face was that look which clings to the memory for ever after, for it spoke of death without its sting.

In the upper division under Miss —— were many cases somewhat similar, but Fisher and Hickey were among the most interesting cases that passed through our hands. Another case of a very different character was in this division.

Sergeant Everett was a ward-master when the hospital was first opened. He had been at the Crimea and there lost his eye. He was discharged from this office for drunkenness, in which he indulged to a fearful extent. He belonged to the Church of England, and the chaplain was ignorant of his propensity, and Sergeant Everett got the right side of him, and the clergyman, being convinced he was a very worthy, religious man, appointed him Scripture-reader.

Everett had the Bible by heart. He could quote texts for an hour without stopping, and his power of talking on religious subjects was very great. He used to go round at night and read the Holy Bible to the soldiers, generally in a state of intoxication. Unfortunately, he contrived to do it at the times the ladies, Sisters, and officers were absent.

One night, however, he was reeling round Lower Stable Ward, Bible in hand, awfully desecrating the name of Christ, when Dr. Temple unexpectedly entered. The doctor immediately reported the circumstance to the chaplain, who of course dismissed him from his situation as Scripture-reader. A week afterwards he was brought into the Lower Stable Ward raving in *delirium tremens*, brought on by his habits of excessive intemperance. He was a fearful case to attend.

He used the words of Holy Scripture in awful blasphemy; he would spring out of bed and knock down the orderlies, and it was with a great effort that the lady and Sister approached him; but they had sufficient power to make him lie still and quiet while they were there: when they were gone, he would recommence, and at night his fearful shrieks would be heard from one end of the hospital to the other. He required much attention, as it was necessary, he should have a great deal of brandy given to him, and it was to be administered to him in very small quantities at a time. Often my hand shook at the glaring look of his one eye as he watched me measure out the brandy. At length he recovered and was invalided home.

To our astonishment, some months afterwards a paragraph appeared in the papers stating he had performed several feats of unheard-of valour at the siege of Sebastopol, which, as he left the camp immediately after the Battle of the Alma, must have been done in his dreams. The paragraph stated he had received presents from both Her Majesty and Miss Nightingale. I am pretty sure he never saw Miss Nightingale at all, and his last statement regarding the ladies at Koulali was utterly untrue.

There were in this ward two Russian prisoners who had been too ill to be moved with the others; they were very gentle and submissive, and the cheerful smile with which they greeted us was somewhat of a relief to the usual heavy cast of their countenances. They were, while in the ward, treated the same as the other sick. They were the lions of the hospital, and a great many sailors and others came to see them, at which they appeared pleased. They talked a great deal to each other, and had a Russian Bible, which they read very constantly. Dr. Temple knew a little Russe, and when he made inquiries after their health in their own language their delight was very great.

This ward, at a later period than this, was principally filled with patients who had been wounded in the camp, and treated in the camp hospitals, and then sent down to Koulali for change of air and nursing before they were invalided home. The lady of the ward often used to remark them great kindness to each other; men who had lost an arm would be seen helping those who had lost a leg to walk, then these in their turn would cut up the food, or help in other ways those who had lost their arm or the use of it as the case might be.

The men were delighted with newspapers, and nine or ten would assemble together while one read aloud, and it was very amusing to hear their remarks on the things going on in the Crimea. They were so astonished and vexed at the attack of the 18th of June: "That was an unfortunate day, we did not gain any honour." One man comforted them by saying, "But no wonder it was not, *as* it was not *men* but *boys* that were driven back and behaved badly."

Some of the men were very clever at needlework, and hemmed dozens of pocket-handkerchiefs and towels to be given to the invalids when going to England, or those going up again to the camp. They also mended hundreds of the blue jackets and trousers, the outer hospital clothing. There was one man six feet two high; he had been wounded in the foot, and was unable to put it to the ground for a long time: he made a dress for an officer's wife in the Crimea, and made besides about thirty or forty sets of mosquito curtains.

We used to laugh among ourselves, and say this was the talented ward, for there were in it an artist and a poet. The artist's name was West, and he drew the picture which forms the frontispiece to the second volume of this work. He was a boy of nineteen, and he had really a talent for drawing figures; the one of the "Sergeant," in the drawing, is an excellent likeness. Of course, the perspective of the drawing has been very much improved since it came out of his hands.

He was very diffident about his drawing, and for some time practised in secret, without ours or the surgeon's knowledge; but at length the admiration of his fellow patients was too great to be kept to themselves; the sergeant too evidently thought it a pity such a likeness of him should be "wasting its sweetness on the desert air," and so one day when the surgeon and lady were going the rounds, and standing by West's bed, the secret was divulged, and how West blushed as he exhibited his performances! When the ice was once broken and he really found we admired his sketches, his pride and pleasure knew no bounds. We supplied him with pencils and paper, and he whiled away many an hour by making sketches of his companions. He was "invalided home."

Another man was in the ward at this time, called Shelley, and he was the poet, and wrote really good lines on the different battles, which I regret I cannot give to my readers.

In this ward too was an orderly, who embroidered a pincushion with beads, and it was really beautifully done; he gave it to the lady of the ward as a token of his gratitude. The men who were nearly convalescent were often set to watch by the bad cases that required constant attention. There was one fine Highlander set to this duty; the patient in the next bed to him was very ill, and Miss H—— gave him in special charge to the Highlander at night. Going the night rounds once she found him lying on his bed, his face turned towards the sick man, and one eye open watching him, ready to spring out of bed at the slightest movement; the lady laughed and said it was just like a cat watching its kitten: this was heard by the others, and the pair went by the names of cat and kitten among their comrades for a long time.

There was another instance of the extreme patience of the men. One young man of the 9th Regiment had been in the attack of the 18th of June; soon after it began his foot was shot off; the spot where he lay was so exposed to the fire of the Russians they could not fetch him in—he lay there the whole day—he tore up his shirt to stop the bleeding, and when the evening fell and they carried him in he was delirious from the agony he had endured from thirst; brain-fever followed, and he had to undergo amputation of part of his leg.

Soon after this he was brought down to Koulali. The movement again brought on fever, and made his leg very bad, and the surgeons found another amputation would be necessary, and they feared he would sink under this. However, it was tried, and he survived. His sufferings were very intense, beyond all expression, but he never murmured. We never heard him even groan except in his sleep, and then his moanings were piteous.

He was nineteen years old. His case was one which required most careful nursing; all the surgeons said, nothing but constant care and nourishment could save him. Great judgment was required in the administration of nourishment and stimulants, and great care also in the preparation of the first, which could not have been done except by the extra diet kitchen. It was pleasant to see his looks of delight when the ladies were waiting upon him, his eyes would sparkle, and many a time did he take the food to please Miss H—— which he would otherwise have turned from in disgust, having completely lost his appetite. At length he recovered, and was able to walk on crutches.

Chapter 10

A Terrible Cholera Case

No. 4 wards were exactly opposite No. 3, on the other side of the Barrack Square; its formation was exactly similar to that of No. 3. No. 4 ward lower was under Sister Anne (of St. Saviour's Home, Osnaburgh Street, an Anglican Sisterhood). No. 4 upper was under Sister M—— B—— This Sister was the one who had been so seriously ill with fever in the winter. She recovered and resumed her duties, and performed them with the utmost zeal and devotion; early in the summer fever again attacked her, and the second attack was even more dangerous than the first. For some days her life was despaired of, but she survived it, and on her recovery the surgeons declared it to be essential she should go home, as it was evident, she could not bear the climate; and to our deep regret, accompanied by Sister M—— C——, she left Koulali on July 2nd.

All the other Sisters of Mercy were fully occupied at this time, and as the number of patients had diminished so as not to render the charge too laborious, both wards were assigned to Sister Anne.

This lady had a good deal of experience in nursing, and gave great satisfaction to the superintendent by her devotion to her work, while she was much and deservedly beloved by her patients. The surgeon in charge of the ward was Dr. Watson; both Sister M—— B—— and Sister Anne spoke in the warmest terms of his skill and attention to the men. No. 4 wards were always kept in beautiful order.

There was a man in this ward named A——. He was in brain-fever and perfectly unmanageable both by ward-masters and orderlies, and even by the surgeon, and they were forced to put on a strait-waistcoat to keep him in bed. Whenever the ladies came near him, he grew calm, a single word seemed, sufficient to compose him, and while they were present, he would lie as still as a child.

A—— was a strong, powerful young man, doubly strong from the fever; his head required shaving, but the operation seemed impossible. No persuasion of doctor, ward-master, or orderly would induce him to submit to it quietly. They told him if he would have it cut quite close to his head it would do as well. No—he raved furiously at the idea. It was night, Sister Anne had gone home and the lady appointed to the night-watch came in, and, hearing of the difficulty, said:

"Now, A——, do let them do it."

"No one shall touch my head."

"That is very unkind of you, A——, when I have come so far to do it for you."

He looked at her and said, "And please, ma'am, have not I come as far to let you do it?" and then, without another word, he submitted while she did cut off his hair.

A—— ultimately recovered.

C—— was another case in No. 4 upper ward; he was for a long time a patient from fever and diarrhoea, but recovered, and after several months of illness was discharged to duty.

A few days after this Sister Anne went up to the hospital at half-past nine one night, as she wished to see a patient who was very ill and decide whether he would require sitting up with. When she entered her ward she was astonished to find the state of confusion it was in. As she stood in the doorway a fearful cry of agony startled her.

What was the matter? C—— had been brought in in a fearful state with cholera.

The information was given her by the ward-master, who was pale with terror and trembled from head to foot. Sister Anne begged him not to show such signs of dismay, reminding him that fear would spread the contagion among the others sooner than anything else.

She then approached C——'s bedside, and when she did so no longer wondered at the alarm of the sergeant and orderlies. It was an appalling sight. His face and hands were of a dark purple, both contorted with cramps, his whole frame convulsed, while at intervals he uttered a low moaning cry, between a scream and groan, scarcely like a human being. Sister Anne afterwards told us that so dreadful was the sight that her first impulse was to turn away, but second thoughts decided her that what he had to bear she could look on.

The surgeon entered and Sister Anne was very glad she was there, for brandy and other remedies were required immediately, and were furnished from her cupboard in the wards. The purveyor's store and the extra diet kitchen were both closed long before that hour of the night, and had they been obliged to send to either of these places for what they required nearly an hour must have been lost, and so violent was the disease and so rapid its progress it might then have been all too late.

As it was, with the means they had at hand for immediate use, and the energetic application of proper remedies with the Divine blessing, although in the two days in No. 4 wards there were six cases of cholera in its most malignant form, they only lost one, and that one had been ill with *delirium tremens* for weeks previous to being attacked by cholera, so that when it seized him not a shadow of hope remained.

There was another case of a man named Ferguson. He came down from the camp in June, and entered No. 4 upper ward, was soon pronounced convalescent, and put on the list for invalided home. The day before the party were to go on board, the surgeon and Sister Anne were going round the wards; the latter observed a marked change in Ferguson, which had taken place in the course of a few hours. Whether his excitement and joy at the prospect of going home had produced fever, or whether he had caught the complaint from someone, we could not tell, but certainly the first symptoms of the fearful disease were plainly visible.

The doctor had stopped at his bedside, as was the custom, to say simply, "You go to England tomorrow," but his eyes fell on the fever-spot on his cheek. He looked at him attentively, felt his pulse, and said—

"Ferguson, I am very sorry, but I cannot decide upon your going to England till I have seen you tomorrow, or at least this afternoon."

Poor fellow, he was so disappointed. With an expression of intense anxiety and sorrow he rapidly assured the surgeon,

"I am quite well today, only weak; much better than I was yesterday. I am quite ready to go."

Sister Anne's heart sank as she listened to his words, for she felt assured his "going home" would not be to England; she was certain that he had no strength to resist the fever now preying on him. After the doctor was gone, in the bitterness of his great disappointment, he wept like a child.

Sister Anne reasoned with him, reminding him how impossible it was the doctor should have any motive for detaining him but for his own good; that he knew how kind the doctor always was to him, and surely he could trust her word. She begged him to keep quiet till the morrow, and not exhaust his little strength by sorrow, for she assured him if he were better tomorrow he should go. He grew calm and satisfied, consented to go to bed and see what tomorrow would bring forth. Next morning when Sister Anne entered her ward her first step was to hasten to his bedside, and it was touching to meet his look of quiet resignation. He said: "Please, ma'am, I don't want to go to England. You were quite right, I'm not fit for it. I am so glad to be here while I am so ill, that you may take care of me as you have done."

Every care was taken, everything that could be done was done, but in vain. He sank rapidly, and in a few days was numbered among the dead.

M—— was another patient in that ward; he lingered for many months in dysentery, which was attended by violent vomiting. This reduced his strength so much that at length he was so low as to be unable to feed himself, and for ten days Sister Anne fed him with a spoon, giving him food constantly in the smallest quantities. He used to entreat her to give it up, saying—

"Please, it's of no use, 'tis only wasting good food."

But of course, she persevered in that and in everything else she thought could possibly conduce to his benefit, and she had the satisfaction to see her efforts, under God's blessing, crowned with success. He quite recovered, and was invalided home. On leaving the ward he came up to her, and, holding out his hand, said,

"Goodbye, ma'am, and God bless you; had it not been for you I never should have been home again."

Among the orderlies belonging to No. 4, was one named H——. When Sister Anne first took charge of No. 4 lower ward, H—— was much, addicted to swearing—so at least she was *told*, for the men were far too respectful to swear in our presence. H—— was also given to drinking.

Sister Anne told him that if he continued in these habits she must ask for his dismissal from the wards. He admitted the truth of all she said as to the sin and disgrace, said he wished above all things to give her satisfaction, and that he would do anything she asked him to do. She said she expected him to give her his promise never to bring brandy into the wards. To this he agreed, and during many months he faithfully kept his word, infringing it only on the occasion of the Battle of the Alma, when much feasting was going on, and an allowance was of course to be made, and he very much conquered the habit of swearing.

Another man, a sergeant, was led to leave off these two habits from Sister Anne's influence. When this man went afterwards to the camp, he wrote letters which cheered the heart of this lady, and which, by her kind permission, we insert.

Camp, Sebastopol, 7th Sept., 1855.

Sister Anne,—I hope you will pardon me for not writing sooner, but the truth is I wrote a letter on the 3rd inst., but it was lost in the tent, and I waited until today thinking I might find it. The bombardment commenced on the 5th. The French opened a terrible fire on the enemy; ours did not commence in earnest until 4 a.m., the 6th inst. On the night of the 5th, we set fire to the large three-decker of the Russians (the twelve Apostles'), and today, the 7th, another large ship set fire to also. The 28th lost one man killed and wounded on the 6th inst. I do not know our loss today as yet, but we are firing very hard all day. We are to have three days' rations cooked in our haversacks tomorrow, and to parade at four a.m., which looks pretty like another attack on the Redan and Malakoff by us. We have no huts up as yet, so I think we will not require them now, for we are all determined to go into Sebastopol this time. We are getting fresh meat three or four times a-week, bread sometimes too, and potatoes occasionally, so we are not so bad off as you think; and, thanks to your kindness, I am better prepared this winter than I was last.

Hoping this little account will not displease you, and you will pardon errors,

 I remain

  Your most obedient Servant,

           J. J——

 Goody was another orderly, and he deserved his name, for he was *good*. Everyone in the hospital knew him for his willing spirit, his sobriety, industry, and constant good humour; he was willing to help everybody, and grumbling did not seem natural to him, but he had such a perpetual grin on his face we thought he must go to sleep with it. Sister Anne talked to him one day about saving his money. He thought it was a capital idea, and he used regularly to bring it to her as soon as it was paid to him. By the time he left the ward it had amounted to a good sum.

 Goody and N—— were quite exceptions to the general rule concerning orderlies; they could be left and trusted very much. Their affection and attention to their patients were remarkable; they were as gentle as women. Sister Anne suggested to them that in the case of patients who were much emaciated it would ease them to be lifted in sheets when their beds were made, and they never forgot the hint.

 There was one orderly in this ward who possessed an unfortunately surly temper. He did not venture to show it to Sister Anne, but visited it upon one of her nurses.

One day when she went to the orderlies' side of the ward requesting him to do some part of the work which was left to him to do, he answered her insolently, and said "she could do it herself." The nurse complained to Sister Anne, who said:—

"This is the second time the complaint has been made to me, and I have warned him that I would not again allow it to pass." She sent notice to the *commandant*. To her astonishment, in a few minutes he appeared at the door of the ward with a sergeant, corporal, and picket of men. The *commandant* expressed his regret any soldier should have spoken rudely to a lady. Sister Anne explained that it was not to herself he had done so, but remarked as the nurses were under her protection it was her duty to see proper respect shown to them.

In this he quite agreed, and trusted she would complain to him at once if any annoyance occurred, that it would be his pleasure as well as duty to assist her. He then asked if she intended preferring a charge against this orderly.

She said certainly not. She only wanted him removed from the ward. This was done (the doctor's sanction having been obtained before the complaint was made), and another man made orderly in his stead. Thanking the *commandant* for his kindness, this formidable affair came to an end.

One morning on going to the ward Sister Anne saw something was wrong with her ward-master. He was one of the best in the hospital, sober and attentive to his duty. He looked very miserable, and came and told her he was a prisoner. She asked, "On whose charge?"

"That of P——, an orderly who had told the *commandant* that Sergeant D—— had been out of the hospital after hours."

She said, "Were you so?"

"No indeed. I was not in my own room, but I was not even out of this division of the hospital; I was in another sergeant's room upstairs spending an hour. The time passed on; I had not told the orderlies where to find me, but they all knew I was in this division."

Sister Anne first satisfied herself as to the truth of this statement. She knew the orderly who had reported him was one who was about to be dismissed that very day for bad conduct, and who had an ill feeling against the sergeant.

She then went to the *commandant*, admitted the sergeant was to blame in not being in his room, but spoke of his general good conduct, the real loss it would be to her, and begged he might be pardoned. The *commandant* as usual listened kindly, but said it was now out of his power to do anything, as it had been referred to the general at Scutari, and D—— must stand a courtmartial.

This was sad tidings for the poor sergeant. He was in despair at the very thought, and begged her to use her influence at Scutari.

She replied that she could do but little there, she feared; she could only testify to his good conduct, and she was sure both his surgeon and staff-surgeon would bear her out, and that she would apply at headquarters, and plead for his return. Beyond her expectations, the case was most readily attended to, and within two days she had the pleasure of receiving intimation that he was set at liberty without a court-martial, that he would have returned to Koulali at once, but that the adjutant having seen him considered him a superior man, and as he wanted a clerk for his office said he wished to retain him for that, and hoped Sister Anne would willingly part from him, as his pay would be treble to what he received as ward-master, and was besides a promotion.

She of course said she would not stand in his way, and there she thought the matter ended, but the best was to come. The following night Sergeant D—— came to the "Home," and begged to see Sister Anne, then told her he could not bear to accept the offer made him without her consent and approval, and that he had told the adjutant so, for that he had received so much kindness from this lady he would rather give up the post than displease her. Sister Anne assured him she had no wish to stand in the way of such an advantage, and was very thankful it had happened. She was much gratified by the good feeling displayed.

The following letters will show more fully the man's character:—

Adjutant-General's Office, Scutari, Nov. 25, 1855.

Sister Anne,—I know you will be pleased to hear from me, and to know how I am getting on in my situation. I can assure you that I have made a good exchange; in the first place I will improve myself greatly, and secondly, I am separated from a few people at Koulali who very probably would get me into another predicament.

I am quite by myself and associated with no one. I am very thankful to you for allowing Sangers to go to my box to take some things out for me. I hope you are quite recovered in health again, and able to attend the 'hospital.' I will content

myself with the hopes of soon receiving a letter from you; and trusting you are in the enjoyment of good health,
>Believe me to remain
>Yours, most respectfully,

P. S.—Please remember me to F—— and ——

>Scutari Barracks, 7th Dec., 1855.

Sister Anne,—I received with deep gratitude your very handsome present, and shall ever feel the warmest sympathy towards you for your many kindnesses to me. I almost feel that I presume too much in addressing a lady to whom everyone looks as a mother, but the poor man, although born in humble life, still has the warmness of feelings in his breast as well as the rich, and with it is therefore, Sister Anne, that I thank you again with all the warmth of that feeling, and shall ever feel it my duty to think upon and speak about you in the circle of my family and friends.

I hope it will be your lot to remain long amongst us, administering the same great comforts and blessings that you have already shown. I feel quite comfortable in my new situation, and I thank you for the expression of your happiness on my promotion in the new line, quite different to the one I had before, although I would have been much happier had I stayed under you, but events occur and we know not until it is too late—but experience teaches us, and I intend to profit by it for the future. I beg of you, then, Sister Anne, to allow me to subscribe myself
>Your most obedient and humble servant,

CHAPTER 11

The Starving System

In another ward in the Barrack Hospital both upper and lower divisions were under the charge of two Sisters of Mercy and two hired nurses. Both wards were under the same medical officer. Dr. ——, a civilian.

There were two civilians in Koulali Hospital, who held about the same position as staff-surgeon, and were much better paid. Their position was an anomalous one; they are nominally under the staff-surgeons and principal medical officer, but pretty much set them at defiance, and sometimes the assistant-surgeons were forced to be under them. The military surgeons of course chafed at the intrusion of these gentlemen, and I only wondered how they bore it with any patience at all, for they certainly did not do credit to the civil branch of the profession.

Dr. —— was a very eccentric person; he had many years previous to the war lived and practised at Constantinople, and had now come out, he said, from a purely benevolent desire to enlighten the military medical staff upon the true mode of treating the sick. We used to wonder whether the £2 2*s*. per day had anything to do with the benevolence.

Dr. —— chose to try experiments on these men. He said their diseases ought to be treated as the diseases of the inhabitants of Turkey were, by starving, quite forgetting the difference in the constitution and habits of the Turks, and also the labours our men had undergone in the camp, instead of spending their days cross-legged on a divan smoking a *chibouque*. But Dr. —— had a profound veneration for Turkey, its habits and customs—he maintained it was the best government and most moral country in the world.

He told us we were sadly wasting our time by not using the privilege of our sex in seeking admission into different *haréems* and cultivating the acquaintance of the Turkish ladies, whose method of managing their households and children was so admirable.

In his ward the most exaggerated form of the starving system was established. How any of his patients existed we could not think—more died in his ward than in any other. Here it is but fair to state that some of the worst cases in the hospital were under his charge, and that the doctor himself insisted his ward was not a healthy one.

Nursing in his ward was a most miserable work: it was the constant witnessing of suffering and no means of relieving it. The ladies one and all declared the impossibility of working under him. The Sisters of Mercy made no remonstrance, and for many, many months patiently and devotedly did they fulfil their appointed duty, and that was one indeed arduous.

The comforts and encouragement which cheered on the ladies and Sisters in other wards failed here. They who had been accustomed to courtesy and cordiality from the army surgeons were met with rudeness and constant hard rebuffs. In other wards if one committed an unintentional error in carrying out, or omitting to carry out, as the case might be, the doctor's orders, we were sure of being treated leniently and being taught how to do better for the future. In this one no mercy was shown to the offender.

The Sisters attached to this ward saw other wards gradually improving while theirs remained in the old state of dirt and neglect; they saw in the extra stores numberless comforts which they knew their men lacked and they dared not procure them for the poor sufferers. They saw the other Sisters and ladies counting numbers of convalescents in their wards, while their task was to watch the slow progress of disease and death in those committed to their care.

The depression of this was extreme—everyone who visited the ward even felt its influence. The superintendent, who of course visited all the wards, often said she could not imagine how the Sisters bore up under their labour; but they never complained, they did all they were permitted to do for their patients, and soothed them with kind and gentle words, and they were not unappreciated.

"Never mind. Sister," said one, "we know you mayn't give us extras as the others do, but we like to see you smile,"

An instance of the doctor's eccentricity may be given. He had a great fancy for putting his men on milk diet; he said all doctors had their *fad*, and that was his. If he had given them enough of his "fad" it would have been different.

In the hot weather it was very difficult to get good milk. There are hardly any cows in Turkey, and the milk was a concoction of goats' and asses' milk, with large proportions of chalk and water (beside it *London* milk would have looked like country cream), and for which we paid the moderate sum only of six *piastres* (twelve pence) the quart.

In hot weather this milk would not stand boiling; we tried heating without boiling, it would not stand that either. The first time this happened was at dinner time, when all the milk turned. A question arose what to send instead of the milk diets; a consultation with the ladies of other wards soon settled the point with them, but the Sisters of this ward dared not give an opinion; so, the lady in charge of the extra diet kitchen sent a message to Dr. —— to know his orders.

He immediately came to the kitchen and said:

"How many of my patients are on milk diet today?"

Glancing at the diet roll, the lady answered, "Eighteen: I was going to send you eighteen pints of rice-milk."

"I will have chicken broth instead," said he; "send me about one pint, or one pint and a half."

"You mean that quantity to each kind of rice-milk which is deficient?"

"No, ma'am," with great emphasis; "I mean one or one and a half pints of chicken broth. That, ma'am, will make four or five ounces' allowance for each man; and you may also send them each one a captain's biscuit," and he then departed.

A group of orderlies were standing by waiting for the ward dinners; when the doctor was out of hearing there was a burst of laughing among them.

"Well, I never!" says one; "if that ain't a rum notion though!—five ounces of chicken broth each for eighteen soldiers! Why 'tis worse than the camp and green coffee."

In the lower ward was a very interesting case named Algeo; he was quite a boy, and was a great sufferer, being covered with abscesses and quite unable to move himself at all; but Sister —— used to say she never saw him without a smile on his face, and when he slept, it was touching to watch the look of calm endurance which was still there.

The orderlies used to carry him out on his bed and lay him outside the hospital, on the shore of the Bosphorus, that the sea breeze might refresh him. All knew he was passing away from earth, and the orderlies and all were kind to this poor sufferer, almost yet a child, whose young life had been so strange and sad; first the battlefield and trench work, then the bed of wasting sickness.

Sister —— tended him with loving care, and he repaid it by his deep gratitude and affection.

An orderly in this ward was called Dick he was quite a character in his way, he was so rough and quaint, and looked as if he was just made to knock down a dozen Russians at once, but Dick was as kind to Algeo as if he had been his own child. Poor Algeo was so fond of him, and it was strange to watch the affection between the rough, hard soldier and the dying boy. His last agony came on, and just before he passed away, he called for Dick.

"Come here, Dick; I want to kiss you, Dick."

And as Dick held him in his arms the boy died.

When the rough orderly told Sister —— of it the tears stood in his eyes.

This orderly was a strange character, he was so remarkably ugly, and was quite aware of the fact and rather proud of it.

"I be the best-looking man in the hospital," he used to say.

One Sunday I called to him as he was passing to take a message for me to one of the ladies. "You are the orderly from No. — they call Dick, I think?"

"Yes, miss, they calls me Dick on week days and Richard on Sundays."

"Dick," said Miss ——, going into his ward to visit a sick man who belonged to the Church of England; "do you know if the chaplain has been here today?"

"I think I see'd him a knocking through the ward," was the answer.

Another ward was occupied by sick when the hospital was crowded, but it was not considered healthy and was emptied as soon as possible and turned into a "detachment ward." Before we describe the other buildings of the Barrack Hospital, we will visit the General Hospital of which we were very proud.

Chapter 12

The General Hospital at Koulali

The General Hospital, Koulali, has been before mentioned. It was originally built as an hospital to the Turkish barracks. Tradition says that on or near to its site formerly stood a chinch dedicated to the Archangel Michael; exactly opposite, on the European side, stood another church of the same dedication, for it was the old Christian belief that the guardianship of all the fortresses and buildings situated on the banks of the Bosphorus was entrusted to the Archangel Michael. It is remarkable that all ancient churches dedicated to St. Michael, not only in the East but in every country besides, are built on hills.

The Turks have one uniform plan for building their hospitals. Koulali was a miniature imitation of the large General Hospital, Scutari, and we admired the mode of building in some respects, and thought that with English improvements the Eastern plan would make excellent hospitals. Koulali General Hospital was a quadrangle, two storeys high. It was built on the slope of the hill so that the main entrance opened on the second storey.

Lovely was the view that one looked upon from the windows of the different wards; hill and water, trees and villages, in one of the loveliest turns of the Bosphorus. In the centre of the quadrangle was a garden which was planted with flowerbeds, and it was the great delight of the convalescent patients to tend them, and cultivate flowers to give to the Sisters and ladies and to adorn their wards with. Here we could see the men, just able to crawl out of their wards, basking in the sun or trying their returning strength in walking on the grass. In the heat of summer, a canopy was erected over the garden.

Bound the quadrangle ran a corridor, which at the time we are speaking of was full of beds, out of which the wards opened. Each ward held about thirty beds. It would be needless repetition to describe them, as their furniture was similar to that of the barrack hospital.

The rooms were square, with no galleries above—a stove in the centre of each. After passing through the upper corridor, we descended the stairs. The lower corridor ran round the building with wards attached. One of these wards was not considered healthy, and was therefore disused when the press of work had ceased. A row of rooms ran opposite the main entrance in the courtyard. Among these were the general kitchen stores, guard-room, and room for storekeepers, servants, &c.

The medical officer first in charge of this hospital was Dr. Hamilton, whose skill and attention to the men were remarkable. Early in the summer he was ordered to the camp, and his loss was severely mourned by the patients, and by the Sisters of Mercy who worked under him. He was succeeded by Dr. Guy.

The nursing of this hospital was under the charge of the Reverend Mother of the Sisters of Mercy, she being of course under the orders of the lady-superintendent appointed by Lord William Paulet, but as the latter could not be on the spot so frequently as she was at the Barrack Hospital, both Miss Stanley and afterwards Miss Hutton wished the reverend mother to be responsible.

The mother had four Sisters, two ladies, and two nurses to assist her. She had long experience in hospital work, and possessed a skill and judgment in nursing attained by few. This hospital from first to last was admirably managed. The medical officers, both Dr. Hamilton and Dr. Guy, and the assistant-surgeons, fully appreciated her value, and there was a hearty co-operation between them. When the means of improvement were placed in her hands, they were judiciously used, and the hospital so improved that it became the admiration of all who visited it, and the pride of the ladies and nurses who worked in it, and we used to call it "the model hospital of the East."

At each end of the quadrangle were apartments; one side was given to the medical officers, the two on the other side to the Sisters of Mercy. One of these formed their community-room, the other their dormitory in which the ten Sisters slept for many months. Out of the community-room opened a very small one, hardly more than a large closet, which formed their oratory. When the soldiers attended their service, they knelt in the outer room. When one of the Sisters was taken ill with fever the medical officers had her removed into a small room in another part of the hospital.

The superintendent deeply regretted the insufficient room given to the Sisters, while we lived in a large house; but the matter of hospital rooms was one over which she had no control.

When the heat of the summer came on the hospital authorities took the matter into consideration, and it ended with five rooms in all being given over to the use of the Sisters.

Visitors to the General Hospital usually visited the Sisters, for they were universally beloved and respected, and they received all who called upon them with the utmost courtesy and sweetness of manner.

Their community-room was a good-sized and pleasant one, and furnished with the utmost simplicity—glass presses round the walls, which formed at once the Sisters' hospital library and free-gift store, as a portion of all free gifts sent to the hospital was always forwarded by the superintendent to the General Hospital; a deal table, a few chairs, and boxes for additional seats, completed the furniture of the room, which, though occupied by so many, was a pattern of extreme neatness, and the warm welcome we ever met there made it a pleasant resting place after ascending the steep hill from below.

Few of us had ever visited nuns before, and we often remarked among ourselves the bright, joyous spirit which pervaded one and all—their work evidently was their happiness, and we often marvelled also at their untiring industry. They never seemed to pass an idle moment, and in their leisure time they were always busy about some needlework or drawing.

The Sisters never left the hospital (except when business took them occasionally to Scutari) but in the evening, when it was considered necessary for their health to go outside the walls and walk on the hills around.

In No. 4 ward, upper hospital, was a poor boy who died at last in a deep decline. He was always craving for food, though it did him no good when he got it. He gave so much trouble to the orderlies, and from disease was so very irritable to them, that they often complained of his ill temper and ingratitude. But, poor boy, one could hardly blame him, looking on his thin, wan face, whiter than the pillow he laid his head upon, asking one minute to be turned this way, then that, then begging for another and another pillow till at last he got so many that the reverend mother, when going her rounds one day, inquired, with great surprise, the reason why this patient had seven pillows.

"Not one too many," said the poor boy; "I don't lay easy anyhow!"

The Sisters were very kind to him, and attended to his little fancies as if he had been a child. He was always asking for sugar-plums and acid drops to moisten his parched mouth.

All these sort of things, sent out by kind friends from England, were of much comfort and were very superior to those made in Turkey. We tried in vain to get acidulated drops and good liquorice both in Pera and Stamboul, and when our English stock was exhausted we were obliged to content ourselves with the Turkish sweets, finding them better than nothing to give to those whose coughs not only kept themselves awake hour after hour, but their poor companions also.

This poor boy was as pleased as a child with some sugar-plums which Dr. Guy himself most kindly bought for him at the little neighbouring village. He used to keep them under his pillow, and the last thing the Sister did for him at night was to make sure he had enough to last till morning. His first request in the morning was generally to have a bit of buttered toast, and to have his wine and water made boiling hot.

It was not at all easy in the early days of the hospital to get either of these two requests attended to without considerable trouble, as there was but one large fire for the cooking of the whole hospital, and that at some distance from the wards; and with so many needing the Sisters' attention it was a long task having to go up and down corridors, waiting perhaps an hour to get a slice of bread toasted and a drop of boiling water, while others were anxiously waiting their return. But as soon as the Sisters had their brasiers this want was supplied, and great was the rejoicing.

None but they who have worked in the Eastern hospitals can imagine the unspeakable comfort a little charcoal brasier and small saucepan became, or what a privilege it was to get ten minutes' use of a fire.

The poor boy died at last, after weeks and weeks of weary, restless suffering.

One thing at this time the patients suffered sadly from was chronic rheumatism, and this often depressed their spirits more than anything else; they felt so hopeless of ultimate recovery, or of ever being "any good again to anybody," as they expressed it.

One tall, fine-looking man, in No. 4 ward, was often seen with the tears rolling down his cheeks. He looked quite well in the face and could walk about, but his left arm was utterly useless from long exposure in the trenches. He was blistered, leeched, cupped, &c., time after time, but it remained immoveable, and he was at length obliged to be invalided to England.

He was evidently so superior to many of the others that we were surprised to see by his card that he was only a private; but one day he related his history. That seven years ago he had been corporal of his regiment, and would probably ere this have obtained further promotion only that he had married without permission. He asked leave to do so of his commanding-officer, but was refused, and, to use his own words, "she and I were both very young and liked our own way, and so as we could not get leave, we married without, and I was degraded immediately and have not obtained promotion since. She died," he added, "a few months afterwards." He related his story with a half-sad, half-proud smile, as if he thought the young wife now in her grave, far away in England—for whose love he had sacrificed his promotion—had been worth the sacrifice.

There was another, an Irishman, suffering from an apparently incurable malady in his limbs. He looked strong and hearty enough to have fought three or four Russians single-handed; but he was also invalided home. His joy at going back to "ould Ireland" was so great that he thought it advisable to drink his own health and those of the reverend mother and Sisters and everyone else in the hospital before his departure, so he persuaded one of the orderlies, who were sometimes open to temptation, to buy him some spirits; and when the reverend mother went in to give the travellers some clothes for their voyage home, she found him showering down blessings upon everyone in such a very excited tone, that, instead of thanking him for those which as soon as she appeared he especially invoked on her own head, she very quietly went up to him, and, taking the large scissors which hung from her girdle, cut from his neck a ribbon, to which was suspended a religious medal often worn by the Catholics.

This silenced him at once: she left the ward with the medal in her hand, and poor Patrick was broken-hearted. He said "he'd have no pleasure in going home now," blamed himself for his folly in sending for the unhappy drink which had caused him this disgrace. In two hours, they were to sail for England—what was to be done? One of the Sisters advised him to go and beg the reverend mother's pardon, and perhaps she would forgive him; he seemed cheered by the hope, took courage and went immediately, begged her very humbly to forgive him this once and he never would take a drop o' drink again till he got to the ould country. Not liking to let him leave the hospital in disgrace, she restored his medal and forgave him with many a word of good advice.

They often wished for a walk on the beautiful hills round the hospital, but Dr. Guy was afraid to give permission, as a few unruly ones might bring trouble on the rest. The innocent as usual had to suffer for the guilty, and that not a little, for it was most tantalising to sit at the gate of the hospital looking out on the lovely country beyond, longing, as the sick so often do, for the flowers and the fresh air, and yet not able to stir a step.

If those who nursed them could have put on the celebrated wishing cap of Arabian Nights notoriety, their patients longing for the green hills would soon have been gratified; but as it was they were forced to console them with the hope of future walks in old England: but it used to fret them sadly, and it was difficult to make them understand that it was at all reasonable for one man to suffer for the fault of another.

The Sisters' influence over the soldiers was very great. Earnest and touching were the blessings poured down on then heads.

"I shall be a different man when I go out of this hospital," said one.

"The prayers of my widowed mother in England will go up to heaven for you," said another.

The Irish were of course vehement in their gratitude, and very amusing besides. "It's myself that's proud to see you again this morning, Sister, and is not it myself that knows who's the best doctors in the hospitals now-a-days?" and some added, "What you gives us is better than all the doctor's stuff."

The convalescent ward, or hospital, as it was sometimes called, contained one hundred and fifty beds. As an ordinary rule, patients from the Barrack and General Hospitals were sent to the convalescent ward to perfect their recovery and gain strength. It was under the charge of a surgeon who lived in an apartment built on to the hospital; a small kitchen and surgery were also attached, so that the patients lived quite separate in every way from the other hospitals.

No nurses were required for this hospital, as all the patients were in a convalescent state. A few were now and then in bed, but if any serious illness arose among them, they were sent back to the other hospitals. The men were, however, visited occasionally by the ladies and Sisters.

We generally went in the afternoon, taking books and writing paper, and envelopes for their letters, and talking to the men, which they always enjoyed, for an hospital life, especially to a man, is a very monotonous one, and they used to appreciate what they called "having a bit of a chat."

The convalescent hospital was much admired; it was kept in beautiful order, and the men looked so well. It was in Dr. Tice's division as 1st class staff surgeon. Dr. O'Callaghan for some months, and afterwards Dr. Carolan, were the surgeons in charge.

Outside this hospital were always to be seen groups of invalids in their blue hospital dresses and white nightcaps, inhaling the fresh breezes from the Black Sea, and watching the vessels going up and returning from the Crimea. The rapidity and numbers of recoveries at Koulali were certainly greatly aided by the establishment and good management of the convalescent hospital.

CHAPTER 13.

Heartbreaking Work

From the first day of our commencing our nursing at Koulali we much wished to have added night attendance as well as day. We felt that the want of this rendered our work imperfect.

During Miss Stanley's superintendence she had deeply regretted that it was impossible with our limited numbers, weakened by illness, and inefficient for the daily toil, to attempt it, except in such a case of emergency as that of the medical officer, whom we nursed at night.

When Miss Hutton had organised the work of her new party, she became anxious to establish it, and though the great sickness and mortality had passed away, yet we felt satisfied for a month or two there was sufficient sickness in the hospital to make this useful and beneficial.

While we were considering the expediency of the plan and the difficulties in its way, and especially whether the medical officers would now like it to begin (they had wished for it in the winter), this point was decided for us. There was a serious case of illness in No. 4 wards; one evening Sister Anne was standing beside the patient considering what she could do more ere she left him for the night, when the staff-surgeon of the division came up and remarked that this was a case requiring watching every hour of the twenty-four. She assented, and added, why is it not done? The surgeon asked if she would sit up? She replied, with all her heart; and she then went on to tell him what a strong wish for the establishment of night work was felt by all, and how gladly we would undertake it.

Arrangements were soon made, and from that time the "night watching" began, and continued regularly for some months. The first night the superintendent took upon herself, that she might more clearly lay down the rules to be followed. She then settled that a lady and nurse should take the office each night. We felt that the nurses could not be trusted without the ladies' supervision, while the ladies needed a companion. If serious cases of illness occurred, which required constant watching, the night nurses were to stay by their bedside; but the ordinary night work was intended for the benefit of those patients who ought not to be left for many hours together without medicine or cooling drinks.

There was a small room opening from our free-gift store, which was a shed in the middle of the barrack yard; this room was used in the daytime by the superintendent to receive persons on business. She gave it up to us for the night work. "We entered it at 10 in the evening, and then went our first rounds.

In each ward there was a table called the Sister's or lady's table; on it we kept books and stationery, flowers, &c. On each of these tables we always found a little book in which was written the Sister's or lady's orders to the night nurse, as, of course, the regular attendants knew more about the cases in their own wards than those merely going in for the night.

It was a rule that one orderly should take it by turns to sit up at night; this, however, grew into the practice of his sitting up one hour, perhaps two, beyond his fellow orderlies, then going to bed in his clothes, which, perhaps, he imagined would keep him awake, but it certainly had not that effect, as he slept as soundly as the rest.

One night the night nurses could not find the Sister's book of directions, and there was a patient who had a blister on and they wanted to know what time it was to be taken off, and other directions about him; so, their only resource was to awake the orderly to know what he had been doing with the Sister's book; the nurse touched, then spoke to him, but no effect, he slept too soundly to be easily awakened; at length she laid her hand on his shoulder and shook him and he opened his eyes, but was some time before he was sufficiently awake to answer her questions. He knew nothing about the blister or the medicine. However, we made him find the book, which he had been meddling with, and then we let him go back to bed.

Generally speaking, we much preferred that the orderlies should be asleep, for sometimes, after having been as we well knew fast asleep till we came in, they would stand up on our entrance, trying to make us believe they had been awake all night; and then they would begin walking about the ward, making such a noise; and they had a peculiar art, known only to themselves, of poking the candle just into a patient's eyes, so that we soon established the rule of their leaving the night watching entirely to us.

The first round finished we returned to our room, and remained there for an hour or two according as our cases required. Some of us were rather frightened at first by the quantity of great dogs who used to rush barking at them from the dark archways of the hospital, and also at the loud voices of the sentries challenging them from the entrance to each ward, with "Who goes there?" However, in a few nights we grew accustomed to it; we used to answer, boldly, to the "who goes there?"—"A friend." Then came the reply, "Advance, friend, and say, all's well!"

We pitied these poor sentries; they had often only just recovered from long illness, and were so weak as sometimes to be quite overpowered with sleep. Knowing that if they were found asleep, they would undergo severe punishment, we always used to rouse them when we found them in this state, and sometimes they would start up, looking very much ashamed of our having caught them, or sometimes—and especially if they had been patients in our wards—thank us for our consideration.

One night we had just reached one of the archways and were about to enter, rather surprised at not having been challenged as usual, when the sentry, quite a boy, who had evidently dropped off to sleep, sprang to his feet and presented his musket, shouting the watchword at the top of his voice. We started back quite frightened.

"Why, sentry!" said the nurse, "are you going to shoot us?"

"Oh, no, miss," said he, lowering his gun, and looking rather ashamed, "but I thought I heard someone coming."

It was rather a break in their monotonous night-watch to see the nurse and lady going their rounds across the barrack-yard to the different wards, carrying hot tea, &c.

In the intervals of our rounds, we occasionally tried to take a little rest, but it was a difficult if not impossible feat. The nightwork altogether was something quite unique in its way, but there was little rest to be found, for our enemies, the fleas, had a decided objection to our doing so; they never approved of it much in the day time, but at night it was altogether against their laws and regulations to allow us to rest for a moment, so we walked up and down and did anything to divert our attention from the misery they caused us.

About twelve o'clock we lighted a fire and set on a kettle to make tea for our next round, and also a little for ourselves. Sometimes we had no wood and had to go foraging for it in the barrack-yard with our lantern, or by the light of the moon, which at times was dazzlingly beautiful, cheered by the songs of the nightingales, who warbled so loudly from the cemetery just above the hospital. When we had collected our wood we returned, lighted our fires, boiled our kettle, and had a cup of tea—all the more refreshing from having had so much trouble about it. The two Russian prisoners in Stable Ward were very grateful for a little tea at night, and told us so by expressive signs.

There were sometimes cases which required unceasing watching, and then someone was required to sit in the ward where the sufferer was lying; sometimes putting a piece of ice into his mouth every five minutes, or a spoonful of wine or beef tea. No words can tell what heart-aching work that nightwork sometimes was, for though those we watched sometimes recovered it was mostly over the dying that we kept vigil in those long, dark wards, lighted here and there by a dim candle, and with three long rows of sleepers.

It was indeed awful to stand by the wakeful, restless sufferer, to mark but too surely the gradual approach of that sleep from which there is no awaking on earth; to see the tossing of the aching head backwards and forwards, from side to side, and be unable to rest it, and to listen to the low moan which alone broke the stillness around.

This was especially the case with the cholera patients: restlessness seemed one of their sufferings. One poor fellow dying of one of the worst forms of cholera was always entreating to be taken away. "Take me somewhere, lift me up, take me away." All through one night this was his entreaty to the lady who watched him. "Pray, pray, take me away, I cannot stop here." She tried every means to soothe him, but in vain.

At last, she softly repeated in his ear the words of some familiar hymns, "*Jesus, Thou our Rest shalt be;*" or, "*There is a happy land far, far, away.*" It pleased him and he lay quiet for a time and dozed a little; but soon awoke with the old entreaty to be moved, to be taken away. His prayer was answered ere next day's sunsetting; he was taken away, and to where "the weary are at rest."

One Scotchman who had lost a leg on the 18th of June was very wakeful at night. Sister Anne, when it was her turn to take the night-watch, remarked upon his extreme cheerfulness. He was in Lower Stable Ward. She said she was glad to see how he kept up his spirits. "Why, ma'am," he said, "it would be impossible not to be cheerful, situated as I am. In the first place I am going home with only the loss of a leg, and I am doing very well at present. I am free from great pain, and I ought to be cheerful and thankful when we are cared for and waited on night as well as day."

We could say with simple truth that many lives, humanly speaking, were saved by night-watching; for, had the care been relaxed, they must have lost at night what they gained by day.

"Oh!" some of the soldiers would say, "it makes the long, long night seem shorter when you come your rounds; when we cannot get to sleep, we lie and watch for the sound of your footstep."

"Will you have something to drink?" we used to say to those we found awake.

"Yes, and God bless you, I am so very dry, my mouth so sore."

And the Irish said they were "just kilt with the drought."

In the summer the nights were oppressively hot, and we often fanned the fever patients with large feather fans, and so soothed them to sleep. If any bad case of serious illness arose in the night, or if we saw any bad symptoms appearing or increasing, we roused the orderly, and sent him for the "orderly officer," this being one of the assistant-surgeons; for they take it in turns to be orderly officer, which is never to leave the hospital for twenty-four hours, and if any emergency arises the orderly officer is always sent for instead of the regular surgeon in charge of the ward.

Occasionally violent storms would occur in the night, the rain would descend in waterspouts like torrents, the gale rise so high that it was impossible to keep our lanterns alight, while the sky was so black, we could not see the glimmering of the lamps at the gateways, and then we really did feel nervous about the challenging, for there were so many Greeks who might have been prowling about the barrack-yard stealing wood or tools, or anything left about, that the sentries were on the alert in dark nights.

However, we never did get shot, and the storms did not occur very often. Soon after we commenced the nightwork the weather grew settled, and it was charming till the intense heat came, and then the nights, though hot, were a relief to the broiling heat of the day.

The moonlight nights were lovely, the surrounding hills stood out so clearly, the barrack-yard was still, and the distant Bosphorus was silvered over—all spoke of rest and quiet, save those many restless sufferers within the wards.

Beautiful was it to watch the morning break and the sun begin to rise—the "*dawning of the morning on the mountains' golden heights;*"—the hills, lit up with rays of gold, the bright-coloured clouds floating in the sky, and making distant Constantinople seem like a city of radiance.

The clear light air raised our spirits, but we were not unthankful when the wards were all astir and our night-watching ended—for we are forced to confess that the vision of bed, and a few hours' sleep therein, began to have more charms for us than the lovely view around us. We took our last round at five a.m. (the orderlies were now wide awake, and able to attend to their patients), and about seven or eight o'clock we walked along the shore, and reached home.

Chapter 14

Shopping at Pera

About this time, we paid one or two visits to Pera for shopping. Pera is never reckoned as Constantinople. "Going to Constantinople" implies in Turkey that you are going to Stamboul or the ancient part of the city.

Our half-hour's voyage in the steamer was very amusing. We embarked either at Candalee or at another village about half-a-mile from Koulali, which was commonly called "Greek town," from the number of Greeks who resided there. Here we had to wait a short time for the steamer which started from Buyukdere, and stopped at these and other villages on the banks of the Bosphorus to take up passengers.

At the pier were always waiting a very heterogeneous mixture of individuals. Turkish ladies in their *yashmacs*, attended by their slaves, women of a lower rank with their bundles and babies, Greek ladies with uncovered heads, their hair wound round in long plaits and adorned with artificial flowers, forming a strange contrast to the others. Men and boys in their crimson *fezs*. The moment the steamer arrived there was a general rush.

Politeness is a branch of education somewhat neglected by the generality of Turkish gentlemen, who mostly push and jostle everyone before them, rush into the cabin and seize upon the best seats, where they immediately begin to smoke, and whether it rain or not never dream of offering them seat to a lady, however much she may need it.

The stern of the vessel is set apart for the Turkish women, and they are confided to the protection of a slave, who keeps a strict eye over his charge. We of course did as we liked, but generally followed the custom of the country, and seated ourselves among the ladies. We took a small Turkish vocabulary and tried to converse with them a little; they were charmed at this, and we always found them extremely affable and anxious to assist us in understanding their language.

How poor do words seem when we attempt to describe the wonderful beauty of that journey down the Bosphorus! Often as we took it afterwards it seemed ever new. The cloudless blue of the sky and the bright sunshine lit up each object with almost unearthly beauty. From Constantinople on the European side, and Scutari on the Asiatic, up to Buyukdere, the Bosphorus is one continuous line of houses, palaces, gardens, cemeteries, mosques, and minarets.

Soon after passing Koulali on the Asiatic side is a palace of the *Sultan's*, painted of a pale lilac colour. This palace is remarkable for its extreme gracefulness and lightness; it looks in the distance as if it were just resting on the water and a blast of wind would blow it away. It was said to be intended by the *Sultan* for the residence of the Emperor of the French, who was at that time expected to visit the East.

On the European side, among the numerous palaces the one nearest the Black Sea is a large pile of building with a beautiful terraced garden and tine trees (an especial beauty in Turkey, as excepting cypresses they are seldom seen). This palace was the permanent residence of the *Sultan*; he came from thence daily to his new palace a few miles lower down to see his ministers and attend to his state affairs.

About three miles below Constantinople, on the European side, is a mosque built of marble, and remarkable even among the many tine ones around for its exquisite carving. It is very small in comparison with the more ancient mosques.

Kuma Ishesmek is a very large village. This town was formerly called Vicus Michaelicus, because Constantine the Great here built a celebrated church in honour of the Archangel Michael which was destroyed, and then again restored by Justinian; after passing this the varied buildings of Constantinople lay spread before our eyes, and the steamer touching the bridge we are at Galata.

The two quarters of the city are connected by a bridge of boats, one end touching Stamboul and the other Pera or the Frank Quarter. Galata and Tophani lie at the foot of the hill of Pera. Galata is the worst part of the city, more filthy than the rest, and crowded by the vilest classes of people of all nations. The steamers all touch at the bridge, and it is necessary to pass through this Galata or Tophani in order to reach Pera. At the extremity of Pera on the summit of a hill, in one of the finest possible situations, stands the principal French Military Hospital.

The Frank quarter has little historical interest; almost the only fact concerning it in former times is the massacre which took place in the reign of Constantine IV., 668.

The emperor gave his two brothers the title of Augustus, and the title without the power raised their ambition. A body of troops took up their cause and approached Galata, making the following extraordinary demand:—

> We are Christians, the sincere votaries of the undivided Trinity; since there are three equal persons in heaven there should be three equal on earth.

Constantine pretended to receive them kindly, and invited them to a conference to discuss this novel view of earthly sovereignty. When they were all assembled, he thought the best way to subdue his brothers' ambition was to show them the bodies of all their adherents hanging on gibbets at Galata.

Such a tale of bloodshed in the far-off times might be told to the traveller in every great city; but to their eyes all traces of such deeds have passed away, and the history of the past seems like a dream; but as one stands in Galata and looks around on those strange old houses, rugged streets, and fierce inhabitants, the time of conspiracy and massacre does not seem so far distant.

After passing through the streets of Galata, crowded with shops filled with the commonest Turkish and English goods and its crowds of sailors, soldiers, and beggars of all descriptions, we arrive at the tower of Galata, from the foot of which is a fine view of the city. This tower was built by the Genoese in 1216, at which time Galata first became a commercial town, for though it is a suburb of Constantinople it is also a town in itself.

The Greek emperors gave the Genoese the privilege of being governed by the laws of their own republic, and they allowed them to fortify Galata with walls and towers which remain to this day. To their disgrace it is recorded that when the Ottoman Army for the last time besieged Constantinople, the Genoese merchants, imagining that they could obtain good terms for themselves from the conqueror, assisted him in his designs. This baseness met with just punishment, and when the Greek empire was laid low the Latin colony also perished. The only remains of the Genoese are a church and monastery of Dominican friars.

Only one mosque is to be found at Galata. There are a great many Greek and Armenian churches. The numerous warehouses in Galata are built of stone to preserve them from fire, but the houses, as usual, are of wood.

One part of Galata is very narrow and particularly crowded; as we were slowly threading our way along a yell was heard, and there appeared coming into the midst of us a huge cart drawn by bullocks and loaded with baggage, violently forcing its way along utterly regardless what became of the crowd. How we escaped being crushed we scarcely knew; we were pushed into a barber's shop, where the barber and his customer just looked up and then continued their respective employments—the one of shaving, the other of smoking—not at all caring apparently whether we were crushed or not. When the *araba* had passed, we proceeded on our way, and though not again placed in such danger, we were often obliged to take refuge in shops when yells or howls warned us a "*hamel*" was at hand.

Hamel is the Turkish for porter. These men seem capable of carrying weights far beyond the strength of an Englishman, though their wretched, distorted-looking figures are very different to the fine stalwart porters on our railways. The *hamels* always look as if they were bent double; on their backs they first fasten a piece of wood, on which they lay their heavy burdens, and they then tramp on caring for nothing that comes in their way, apparently as insensible to all around as if they were beasts of burden. One can hardly believe they are human beings, and the frightful yells they utter help to increase this feeling. Now and then, from extremity of fatigue, they halt and stooping down to the ground rest their burdens and themselves, then on they push again with renewed cries.

Beggars abound in Constantinople, and they present pictures of squalid misery, dirt, rags, and disease, unequalled in any city in the world. They are sights from which one involuntarily turns away. At Tophani there is a market for fruit and vegetables; among the former there were thousands of melons; they are nearly all water melons and taste like cucumbers. The heaps of fruit and vegetables are very well arranged and have a pretty effect. In the centre of the market-place is a beautiful fountain; it is of white marble, the roof slopes, and it is decorated with scriptural devices and sentences from the *Koran*.

Most people embark here for Scutari and the villages on the Bosphorus, preferring it to the din and bustle that goes on at Galata bridge. Tophani is quite bad enough in this way, but a few degrees better than Galata. Weary work is it after passing through Galata to climb the hill of Pera, especially on a hot summer's day; no shade to be found from the broiling sun. There is no pavement, or worse than none, for stones intended for paving are scattered about in all directions as though, as someone described it, they had tumbled suddenly out of a cart.

At the summit of the hill, we found ourselves in the "*Grande Rue*." Here are the shops and the hotels. The *Hotel d'Angleterre*, generally spoken of as *Missiri's*, which can be known at once by the group of English gentlemen lounging about, whose costumes are of an extraordinary description—each one appearing to adopt something perfectly unique. An English gentleman is seldom seen in Pera without a white covering on his hat, or a white scarf round his wideawake.

Then come the Russian and Dutch embassies, and further on, beyond the extreme end of the "*Grande Rue,*" the British Embassy, and beyond that again, in a commanding situation, the principal French hospital. In the "*Grande Rue*" stands the Russian Embassy—a very fine building now occupied as a French hospital.

The shops in the "*Grande Rue*" are kept either by French, or Greeks who can speak the French language. Here can be bought inferior French or English goods at an enormous price. A curious spirit of independence exists among the Pera shopkeepers. They do not in the least care whether you buy or not, and if one walks in and asks for a dress, one or two perhaps are laid down for your inspection, and if you do not like them you may go without. It is in vain to point to others you may see in the distance, you will not have a nearer view.

The French as well as Greeks always ask exorbitant prices for their goods, and expect to be beaten down, taking at last nearly double what the article would be worth at home. Of course, the immense influx both of French and English into Pera, owing to the war, has much increased this spirit of independence and extortion among the shopkeepers, as they are pretty certain of finding customers for their goods sooner or later, and many to whom money is little or no object.

The general idea of the shopkeepers in Turkey is that the English are extremely rich, and only want an opportunity of spending their money which they have no objection to afford them. Another annoyance is that one can seldom get two articles of different sorts in one shop; you buy a dress, and want ribbon or braid to match—you must go to another shop. A pair of gloves, you must go elsewhere; blonde or net, they do not keep it, and so you are sent about from one shop to another till your patience is fairly exhausted. A common reel of English sewing cotton is a luxury rarely to be obtained.

Most of the English considered going to Pera a sort of punishment. It was indeed very fatiguing, but we thought still there was much enjoyment. The "*Grande Rue*" was like an ever-moving picture. The narrow street was crowded with foot passengers, every now and then driven into doorways to save themselves from being run over by horsemen, Turkish carriages, or "*hamels*."

Walking along, one met with every imaginable costume—now a Turk, then a Greek, next a French lady in full Parisian costume, French officers, English and Sardinian *ditto*, English, French, and Sardinian soldiers; a *pasha* on horseback, with his train; a group of Turkish women; another of Greek ladies; a Greek priest in flowing robes, long beard, and square cap; a Greek Catholic priest, distinguished from the other by the black gauze veil thrown over his cap; an Armenian priest in dark brown robes; a group of French clergy; an English chaplain; a *Soeur de la Charité*; a group of English sailors—so went the scene, so ran the din of many tongues.

Passing up the "*Grande Rue*" we reached the British Embassy, which is a large mansion standing on an eminence and commanding a magnificent view; just at its foot lies a Turkish cemetery, with its attendant cypresses. The Golden Horn, the first windings of the Bosphorus, the Sea of Marmora, the distant range of mountains, Scutari, with its hospitals, all lie spread before the eye that gazes out of the embassy windows.

Strange indeed must it have seemed to its occupants looking down from their palace over the fair view before them upon the abode of suffering, where the pride of the land they represented were dying of pestilence. What wildest romance could have imagined the change a few months had brought? Once no bitter feelings of a nation's humiliation mingled with the sight—but now, who shall from that residence ever gaze unmoved on the spot where so many British soldiers have suffered—on the ground where so many have lain down to their last rest?

The embassy is a fine building, standing in grounds of its own. On our return from thence we were proceeding down a narrow street which led into the "*Grande Rue*," when the dismal sound which the Greeks make in chanting struck on our ears. We saw a procession in the distance, and we squeezed ourselves against the walls as best we might to let it pass. Boys bearing tapers came first, then priests; followed by a bier, on which was laid the body of a young girl.

The corpse was uncovered, that all might gaze on it, and strewn over with flowers; the pale, marble-like beauty of her face contrasted with the freshness of the roses, a chaplet of which crowned her head. A few hours only has she ceased to breathe, yet so soon are they bearing her to her last resting-place on earth; and the young face, from which life has but just fled, must in so sadly brief a period be shut out from the gaze of those who have loved it. It is this necessity for almost immediate interment after death which makes it so doubly painful to witness it in Turkey.

Illness, death, and burial follow each other in such rapid succession, that to the survivors it must often seem like a dream rather than a reality, that the joy of their homes and the sunshine of their hearts are gone from their gaze for ever in this world. More boys with tapers followed the bier, and then came the mourners. As they passed into the distance the chant sounded like a wail, and strangely indeed in that crowded city on that bright summer's day, did the passing sight of the calm face of the dead fall upon one's heart.

Descending from Pera we took the turn leading to Tophani, and thus escaped the disagreeables of passing through Galata. At Tophani pier (if such a name can be given to the construction of a few half-broken planks) we found many *caiques* lying, and were assailed as usual by the shrieks of *caidjees*, some pulling one's cloak to induce one to get into their *caique*. We were thankful when our interpreter had settled the question of fares, our next feat was to jump from the crazy pier into the middle of the *caique*, so as to keep the balance of the boat—then to settle down on the cushions at the bottom, and so lying full length, the *caidjee* pushed off and wound his way marvellously among the multitude of other craft which completely covered the water round the pier.

This was no easy matter owing to the enormous quantities of boats and *caiques* surrounding us. It has been estimated that the number of *caiques* plying on the Bosphorus counts from eighty thousand, and upwards.

At last we were free and swiftly we glided onwards past the great ships lying at anchor off Tophani—past palace and mosque and garden down the sunny Bosphorus, watching the different *caiques* as they glided by—now filled with Turkish women, their bright eyes glancing at the strangers from beneath their *yashmacs*—now a boat full of laughing Greek girls—now a grave Turk alone with his *chibouque* and his slaves—now one full of European gentlemen, whose costumes were quite as *remarkable,* and bore almost as little likeness to home as the Turks themselves.

"*Sooltan, Sooltan,*" says the *caidjee.* We were passing his new palace, and he was about to enter. Our *caidjee* rests on his oars respectfully till the monarch disembarks. The Royal *caique* touches the marble steps, the iron gates are wide open, the twelve rowers, all dressed in white, stand up, their hands hanging down straight by their sides—the attendants do so likewise.

No one assists the *Sultan* to rise or step from his *caique.* The slight, feeble-looking man walks slowly up the marble steps and pathway leading to his palace. His loose great coat and crimson *fez* do not distinguish him from a *pasha*. He opens the door himself and walks quietly in; not till he is fairly out of sight do the attendants move from their statue-like quietude and prepare to follow their master. Such is Turkish court etiquette.

Now we glide on, and the sun has gone down and the delicious breeze from the Black Sea blows upon us, and we are silent and look around. The last rays of the setting sun are lighting up for a few last minutes mosque, dome, and minaret, and village, and the many sombre groups of cypresses on either bank, and in the distance the hospital of Koulali, the bright red colour of its walls standing out against the dark hills beyond.

And now the sun sinks below the horizon, but we are not at home, for the current is strong, and our *caidjees* begin to pull more vigorously, for they have a sort of superstitious dread of being on the Bosphorus after nightfall, and they give us to understand very emphatically in their broken English that they shall expect more "*backshish*" on their arrival than they agreed for at Tophani, pointing up to the sky and saying,—

"Plenty dark."

"No plenty sun."

"English, *madama, bono chok bono.*"

"No *bono Russe*, no *bono* Greek"

"Turk *bono*, English *bono*; English, *madama*, plenty money, plenty sovereigns—*caidjee chabouk* home, *madama*, give him more shillings."

"*Chabouk* (make haste), then, *caidjee*," we reply—"sixpence more, *caidjee; shudi, shudi* (quick, quick).'"

And now the moon rises and bathes all around in its shadowy light, and we are thankful that earth is so beautiful; and now our journey is ended—the *caique* touches the threshold of our "Home on the Bosphorus," Georgi and Demetri, our Greek boys, fly down to welcome us, and thus our day's shopping in Pera is ended.

CHAPTER 15

Soeur Bernardine

Even with our interpreter's help we still found great difficulty in shopping at Pera; especially at this juncture when we were obliged to buy so many things for the men, and did not know where to find them, as they were things out of the common way. Papafée did not always know the price; of course he never confessed his ignorance, but only shrugged his shoulders, said it was great nonsense to want them, and let the Greeks cheat as they chose.

Soeur Bernardine, one of the French *Soeurs de la Charité*, hearing of our difficulty, offered either to do commissions for us, or to accompany us through the streets of Pera and show us the right shops. She had been many years in the East and spoke Turkish. We availed ourselves of her kindness, and one day under her escort we traversed the streets of Galata and Pera to learn the best shops to go to: *Soeur* Bernardine knew the right price to be given for everything. She went up and down the extraordinary streets seeking for the treasures of useful, not ornamental, kind of baskets, darning cotton, and worsted stockings (the English kind of the latter are most difficult to procure in Constantinople), gill measures too we sought and *found* with her aid, and many cooking utensils.

We procured a store of treasures in that day's shopping, and valuable information as to the shops at which to buy, and the prices to give, from *Soeur* Bernardine. As we walked along the crowded streets we met among the motley throng, as usual, many French officers and soldiers, and all drew back to let *la Soeur* pass, and taking off their hats bowed as if to a lady of noble rank; for throughout the French Army exists a deep affection and gratitude to their *Soeurs*, and well may they have it towards those who have followed wherever the flag of France has gone to strife and bloodshed. Wherever her sons have lain languishing on beds of sickness, when home and friends were far, one comforter was ever at hand, one well known form hovered by their side—*la Soeur de la Charité*.

Whenever the French Armies for the last 200 years have gone out to battle, as surely as they take with them weapons of war and destruction, skilful generals to lead them to victory, gallant hearts to fight, so surely do they also take a gentle holy band of *Soeurs de la Charité*; and amid those rough soldiers and among those scenes of horror and distress the *Soeurs* move fearless and unharmed. Around them is a shield which insult dares not touch. As safe on the battlefield, or in the hospital tent, or the "ambulance" in some foreign town are they as in their convent home; the "wards of the hospital or the streets of the city are their cloisters, hired rooms are their cells, the fear of God is their grating, and a strict and holy modesty their only veil." No wonder the Frenchman pays them such respect and honour, for they are worthy of it tenfold.

After we had finished our shopping, and were very weary, *Soeur* Bernardine begged we would come and rest at their convent. *La Maison Notre Dame de la Providence* is situated in Galata, it is not far from the British and French Admiralty Offices, but though an extensive building and standing close to a Catholic church, it is in such a narrow, dirty little street that, unless guided there by someone knowing the way, one might wander about for an hour without discovering it. It stands in the midst of the Frank population of the city, its most filthy and abandoned haunts.

Arriving there, over a large door is written, *Maison Notre Dame de la Providence, Ecole des Soeurs de la Charité*. Raising the knocker, the door opened by a pulley from within, and we entered. This convent is in itself a wonder; on one hand is the reception parlour, which is constantly thronged. Persons of all nations come here to ask information on various points; French officers come about their soldiers' wants. Here throng the poor of all descriptions. Everybody in trouble, distress, or perplexity, seems to come here to be relieved.

We pass a little further on into the great store-room, where biscuits and wine and such like articles are dispensed from this house to the "ambulances;" the ambulances are a sort of out-stations for the *Soeurs de la Charité* established near to each hospital; a certain number of *Soeurs* under a *Supérieure* are sent to these stations, and are supplied from this convent with stores for their patients. This convent is the *Maison Mère* for all the *Soeurs* scattered about the Turkish empire; here they return when they are ill for rest and nursing. There, are 100 *Soeurs* in this convent, exclusive of those sent out, and women of eight different nations are in the community.

Leaving the store-rooms we visited the schools, which contain many hundreds of children, of as many countries as are gathered together at Constantinople—which are almost all the countries of the known world—and the children of this strange gathering are all taught one common faith, gathered into one fold. It was a wonderful spectacle to look on the various faces of the little maidens, the blue-eyed German, and dark Italian; the cunning face of the Greek and stolid look of the Turk. Next to the school we passed through the courtyard, where the children play.

A door opening from this admitted us into the adjoining church, which belongs to the Lazaristes Fathers. It was very plain and possessed no ornament worthy of note, save one or two fine paintings. Ascending stairs we next visited the *Soeurs'* dispensary, which is kept in the most perfect order. The *Soeurs* are trained to make up medicines, and this is a most important branch of their work in Turkey, as they are the only doctors for large numbers of the poor, and among the poor exists a quantity of disease far exceeding any other city of the size and population of Constantinople.

Ascending another flight of stairs, we came to the orphans' dormitory. This we found in beautiful order; long rows of little white beds, and at each end, curtained off, was the simple bed of a *Soeur*, who by night as well as day guarded her orphan charge. Higher still—we sighed at the number of stairs—and we found the orphans—one hundred of them, such a happy-looking set, sitting at work in a spacious room, *Soeurs* with them of course.

At our request they sang a hymn. We distributed some sweetmeats among them, which gave great delight. The orphans do a great deal of needlework towards their own support; they also dress dolls in the different costumes of the country for sale, and other articles of fancy work which can be purchased in the parlour below.

The *Soeurs* have a boarding-school for girls, of a higher rank than the day-school. There was not sufficient room for this in the convent, in consequence of the number of *Soeurs* attending the different military hospitals, and the boarding-school had been moved to a house in Pera. The *Soeurs* serve six or more military hospitals in Constantinople.

When we had seen the orphans, we had not even then reached the last story; another flight yet and we found the children's chapel. It is merely a room set apart for this purpose, and tastefully ornamented, though with great simplicity. Stepping out from the chapel we found ourselves on the house-top, which forms a broad terraced walk, and—oh, what a panorama was before us—what pen could describe it? The curious maze-like streets of Constantinople lay at our feet.

We were too distant to see their drawbacks, we only saw the picturesque. There was the bridge of boats, with its thronging multitudes, whose forms looked shadowy in the distance. The Golden Horn and its shipping, the distant minarets of Santa Sophia, Sultan Achmet's mosque, and many a mosque and palace, besides cypress groves, the grand seraglio, and the beautiful rounding of Seraglio point, the blue Bosphorus, the great cemetery of Scutari, the hospitals on the cliff, the Sea of Marmora, the distant chains of mountains, where the eye strives to distinguish the faint outline of Olympus. All this the eye can gather in from any eminence in Constantinople.

The *Soeur's* possessing no grounds to their house come here to catch the fresh air. Here every August the *Soeurs* make, according to their rule, a week's retreat, and those *Soeurs* from the different ambulances change and flock in here for this end, and they spend much of their time on this quiet house-top. *Soeur* Bernardine said, in her pretty broken English—

"It is the time we love the best of all, for then we come here and we have nothing to do but to pray and think of God. Last year," she said, "I was here, I was so happy, but, alas! the cholera broke out at Varna and they sent for us in haste, and I and some more had to go so quickly."

The *Soeurs de la Charité* are those whom I mentioned as having met on board the *Egyptus*. They were founded two hundred years ago by St. Vincent de Paul, a man of whom it has with justice been said, he "did more good in his single life than all the *philosophers* the world ever saw." He thought that to effectually relieve the sufferings of the poor—besides the religious orders established for the relief of particular kinds of distress—there should be an order of women taken themselves from the poor, who would be thus inured to the hardships they had to endure; and he ordained that they should wear the peasant dress of the period, that they should be sent to nurse the sick at all times and in all places where they might be required as well as educate young children.

Persons wishing to enter this order were to pass five years at least in the noviciate, after which they were allowed to take the threefold vow of obedience, poverty, and chastity, but this vow was to expire every

25th of March, and to be renewed or not at the *Soeurs'* own will. No instance, we believe, has ever been recorded of a *Soeur*, after having passed through the noviciate, withdrawing. St. Vincent do Paul died in 1660, but his work lived on. He called his daughters the servants of the poor, but the people saw their deeds of love and they named them *Soeurs de la Charité*.

From France, its birthplace, this wonderful order—wonderful in its extreme simplicity—spread into all lands. They number now eleven thousand. Ladies of high rank, even princesses have laid down their rank and wealth and entered the lowly order of the daughters of St. Vincent, but the greater mass of the *Soeurs* is composed of the class for whom St. Vincent intended it—the women who in England are hospital nurses and schoolmistresses.

This is the order which made the *infidel* Voltaire exclaim, that if anything could make him believe in Christianity it would be such deeds as those wrought by the *Soeurs de la Charité*.

In the din of the French Revolution, even in the Reign of Terror, the *Soeurs* won respect from those fiends in human form. In the Peninsular war one town was constantly taken and retaken by the French and Spaniards. In this town was a convent of *Soeurs de la Charité*. Whichever army occupied the town they sent sentinels to guard the convent, for the influence of their gentle deeds of love triumphed over the bitter animosity of war.

The mission of *les Soeurs de la Charite* in Constantinople was founded in the following way. Fifteen years ago, a German lady came to Paris and sought to enter the order. On inquiry she was found to be above the age at which the novices are received, which is either twenty-eight or thirty. The disappointment was great, for it was the wish of her heart, and at length the superiors of the order agreed to receive her should she be willing to endure the test they would put to her. They wished to found a house in Constantinople, they said, would she go there with one companion, establish a school, and so make their footing good? She consented.

Fifteen years ago, Constantinople was a very different place to Constantinople now. The Christian's life then was one, in outward things, not much unlike that of His Divine Master—pelting with stones in the street and other insults were the portion of these holy women. They persevered. *Soeur* Bernardine (for she was the lady we speak of) learnt the Turkish language, established a school—*Soeurs* came from France, and she entered their order.

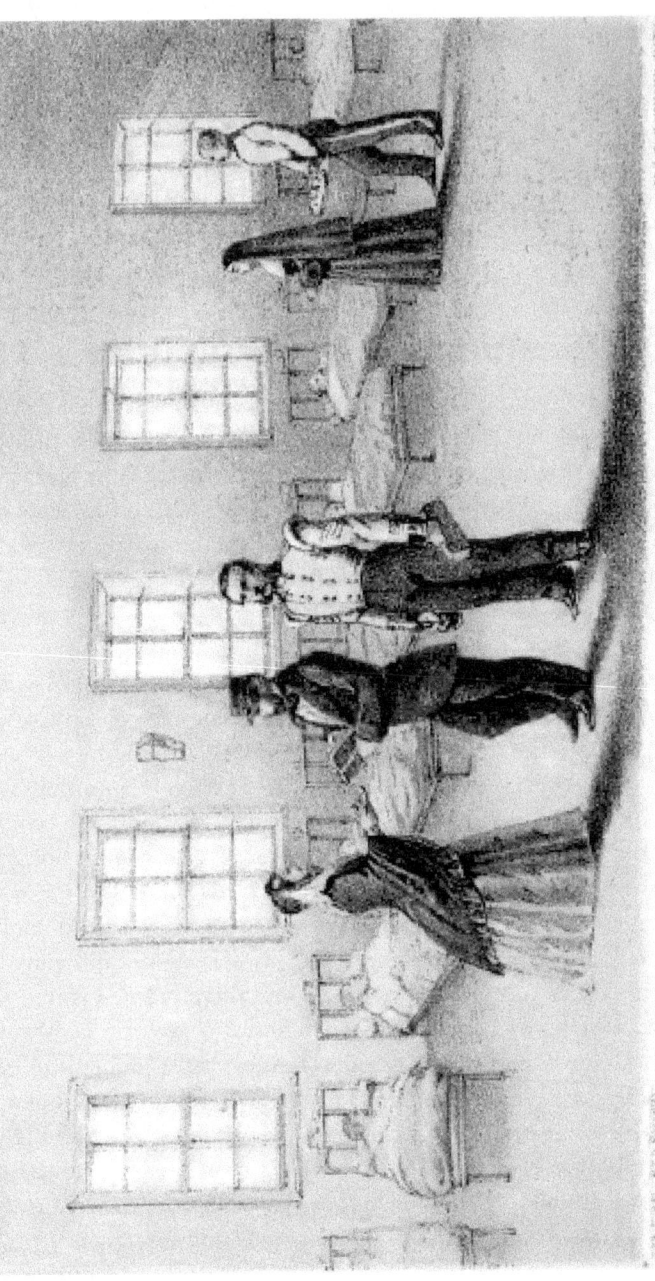

LOWER STABLE WARD KOULARI BARRACK HOSPITAL.

London Hurst & Blackett, 1858.

Sweet *Soeur* Bernardine! my memory loves to linger upon her. We shall never meet on earth again, but never shall I forget that saintly face, or that winning, loving manner, which spoke so plainly of the well of love within her heart. The toil the *Soeurs* undergo shortens their lives; many have died of fatigue during the present war—four at the convent in Galata within a few weeks of each other. A lady who had been boarding at the convent told me she never witnessed such peaceful deathbeds. Humbly but joyfully, they went to Him they had so loved to serve on earth.

CHAPTER 16

Difficulties and Impossibilities

Up to this period the improvements in the hospital had been slow and unsatisfactory, and were owing more to the merciful cessation of death and suffering than to any exertions on the part of the authorities; to this we must except the medical staff, who, as far as our knowledge went, exerted themselves to provide all the remedies and create all the improvements they could consistently with the routine of their work; but this routine was so rigid that many necessary improvements fell short of its scope.

The two departments of the army who have most concern with its hospitals are the medical and the purveying ones, the commissariat belonging only to the army in the field. Up to May, 1854, the purveying department continued in a most inefficient state. Requisitions on the stores for necessary articles were constantly dishonoured, while anything out of the common routine was never to be thought of.

Of course, in Turkey there were all sorts of difficulties in the way of procuring the usual comforts for the sick, and up to this time everyone, excepting the *Times* commissioner, looked upon a difficulty as an impossibility. It was difficult to get wood, therefore it was impossible to have tables or benches. It was difficult to get iron bedsteads, therefore the men must lie on wooden trestles. It was difficult to get good washing done, so it was left to go on as it best could. Cooking utensils were scarce and dear, so the food must be cooked without: the ladies' hands were crippled by being wholly restricted to the use of the articles furnished by the diet-roll, and all deficiencies were to be supplied by our free gift store, which was small and uncertain.

We continued to buy many things ourselves, kind friends sent us presents also; but we felt the painful uncertainty of this, and we also felt this was not the way in which the Army of England should be relieved. Private charity had flowed forth in our emergency, but it should not be overtaxed. The government of England ought to be the source from which it should permanently come. When Mr. Robertson, the new purveyor in chief, came into office, this was realised. The purveying department was soon in a very different state—in working instead of idling order. What was required in the hospitals was procured without delay. First came iron bedsteads and hair mattresses; next tables and benches; a sufficiency of tins for the men's food to be eaten out of.

Other improvements followed. The hospitals assumed a different aspect; now, indeed, were English soldiers treated as they deserved. The just complaints began to be hushed; not that the improvements were wrought at once or without labour and difficulty; but Mr. Robertson was a person determined to overcome obstacles, and who went simply and straightforwardly about his business.

It was now we gained possession of the charcoal brasiers, of which incidental mention has been made. These treasures deserve a more particular description. They are small iron tripods, holding a few pounds of charcoal. They are very difficult to light, and the fire can only be kept alive by being placed in a draught. In the winter, as we have described, we did all our cooking for ten days upon them, but those we then used were borrowed for the emergency.

All the ladies and Sisters complained of their not having any fire to go to if they wanted, as so often happened, to make a cup of arrowroot, or warm some wine or water, &c., and it was so tiresome having to send so frequently to the diet kitchen for every little thing: first, it was such a long way off, and in consequence the fetching and carrying took up more than double the time it ought; and secondly, the workers in the diet kitchen found it almost impossible to keep it in order if orderlies and nurses dropped in at all times asking for every imaginable article, so that a charcoal brasier for each ward had long been one of the objects of our ambition, and now we had but to write requisitions for them and they were procured immediately. They were placed in the lobby of each ward, both that they might have a draught and also not be an annoyance to the patients.

At night we used our "Etnas." These valuable helps to those who nursed the sick were brought from England by the ladies—they were given by kind friends in England as a last thought for our own comfort should we be laid up. Little did the donors imagine the vicissitudes their Etnas would go through in an Eastern campaign till they were fairly battered out.

Before the charcoal brasiers arrived, they were constantly used, but of course the spirits of wine required to light them made them rather an expensive luxury. Still, they were our night companions, and many a little comfort did they enable us to give to our poor men, to whom they were also an extreme amusement. They would sit up in bed sometimes to watch us boiling an egg or some arrowroot in one of them, saying one to another—

"Ain't that a little beauty, now? It's as handsome a little pot as I've see'd since I left England. I wish we'd had it in the trenches; there were no such things as them up there." Poor fellows, they were easily amused, and it was a real pleasure to us to hear them laugh.

The next good thing that happened was the construction of the ladies' ward-rooms, which was simply dividing off in each ward a small space by means of canvas screens in which were placed two or three chairs and a table; this was a great boon to the ladies, who could thus occasionally take a few minutes' rest, which before they could not obtain except by leaving the hospital and returning home.

The introduction of canvas screens into the wards was a great improvement. Now the delirious, or cholera, or dying patients could be screened off from the others. Before this the sight of the very terrible cases often had a sad effect on their fellow patients.

The fruit season had commenced, and every day the *caiques* loaded with fruit dashed past the windows of our home. Strawberries were first, through Mr. Stow's kindness, introduced into the wards. Mr. Robertson said the government ought to provide them, and we had as many as we required.

The strawberries were very fine, though they did not seem to us to possess the flavour of English ones. There were quantities of melons brought in *caiques* for sale, but this was a fruit very seldom wanted in the hospital, and the men did not like green figs, of which there were quantities; grapes followed, and they were much appreciated by the fever patients.

Then came the astounding news that the soldiers were to be supplied with pocket-handkerchiefs. Up to this period none were given in the hospitals but from the free-gift store, and it used to be perfectly absurd to hear the ladies begging for them from their superintendent. They were so prized by the men, especially when they were of some bright colour: in fact, with very few exceptions, the men highly appreciated anything which conduced to habits of cleanliness and neatness.

One day a box for me arrived from England, upon opening which I found the contents to be writing paper with views of the war—that published by Messrs. Rock Brothers, Walbrook. A kind friend had sent me a large quantity, and Messrs. Rock themselves added a present of more. Its arrival created a great sensation in the hospital. The ladies and Sisters begged hard for a share. They could not all have it. I gave some to the General Hospital and the rest to the Barrack.

It was a great pleasure to distribute them. I spread one of each different view out on the table, and begged the soldiers to make their selection. Everybody who could walk at all crowded round the table. Orderlies and sergeants left their work to have a look, and even the medical officer was attracted by the crowd and came to look and admire. The different views were carried round to the patients in bed. The business of choosing took a long time. Each wanted some scene in which he had formed a part.

Some had been with Colonel Chester when he so gallantly led on the 20th; those who had been in the Battle of the Alma wished for that; those who had been at Balaclava another; while those again who had fought at Inkermann another. Some had seen General Strangways die, and wanted his last scene; others were less warlike and chose the pretty views of the valley of the Alma before and after the battle, while the comic pictures were not without their share of admirers.

One sergeant was particularly struck by the "Fresh Arrivals"—two young officers fresh from England, in all the pride of new uniforms and polished boots, meeting an old campaigner on a mule who had been out foraging for the mess-table and was bringing home his purchases. The sergeant held this up for the admiration of his comrades, and there was a shout of laughter instantly raised.

I much wish my friend and Messrs. Rock also could have seen the extreme pleasure these gifts were the means of giving—the delight it gave the soldiers to write home on these sheets of paper, or how they were treasured up and compared with each other day after day, and many a tale did the pictures elicit as they brought back more vividly to mind past scenes of Alma and Inkermann, &c. When I wrote home, saying how grateful I was for the present, and how much it had been valued, the same friend sent another packet, which shared the fate of but too many other kind offerings and *was lost,*

Stationery was very much prized; all we had was supplied from our free-gift store, and up to this period had been very scarce, but about this time we had a great deal sent out to us and could supply the demand sufficiently. Now that we had plenty of tables in the ward, we had a store of paper, envelopes, pens, and ink lying on it for all, and in some wards a box to receive the letters, which was emptied on Sunday and Wednesday evenings, and the letters carried home by the ladies and sorted; those to the camp did not need a stamp, those for England were stamped by the chaplain, to whom we gave them.

Extraordinary were the directions and spelling that used to occur in these letters—we often wondered how they ever reached their destination. One very common direction to the camp was "Sebastopol, Russia, in Turkey."

There was one great trouble which we began to feel at this time—namely, the conduct of the hired nurses. We had indeed been tried by this from the beginning, and several, as I have mentioned, were sent home for bad conduct; but still the distress around them and the frequent sickness among their own numbers kept some sort of check upon them, and after some had been dismissed for bad conduct and others from sickness only two remained when the new party arrived on April 9th.

The hospital costume in which Miss Stanley's party left England was worn alike by ladies and nurses, which was intended to mark the equality system, but soon after beginning hospital work, we found it impossible to continue wearing the same dress as the nurses, and therefore discontinued it. When the new party arrived, to our dismay we found that the home authorities had not thought well to learn experience from those who had to struggle with difficulties on the spot; they still held to similarity in dress, and the ladies and nurses all wore the government costume. When we received them at Koulali we expressed our surprise and vexation at the mistake, and our conviction that the ladies would very soon follow our example and make a distinction in dress between themselves and the nurses, and the event proved our expectations correct.

The ladies soon found it was necessary for their own comfort and for the good of their work that in every possible way the distinction should be drawn. None but those who knew it can imagine the wearing anxiety and the bitter humiliation the charge of the hired nurses brought upon us, for it should be remembered that we stood as a small body of English women in a foreign country, and that we were so far a community that the act of one disgraced all. After this period, it is true, we had no longer to encounter the hardships some had endured in the winter, but as long as the work in the East lasted so long were there difficulties to be surmounted and trials to be borne of no common character.

On April the 21st, a second party of three ladies and seven nurses joined us. They had travelled under the escort of Mr. Wallace, a clergyman of the Church of England. Immediately on their arrival he informed the lady superintendent that one of the hired nurses had behaved so badly on the passage out she ought to go home; it was fixed she should return by the next ship that left.

Before the party of nurses, he had escorted out went to their work, Mr. Wallace wished to address a few words to them, but upon their assembling in the sitting-room one of the number, Mrs. ——, declared she did not wish to hear it, as she did not intend to stay. No, the life was "different to what she had expected"—she had been two days in the East—and the nurses "were an ungodly set she could not live among. She was a Christian, and Christians must not live among the ungodly."

Upon inquiry we discovered that Mrs. ——'s husband was a bandmaster, that she had come out intending as soon as she reached the East to leave the service of the government and join him, but on her arrival, she found he had been sent home, and now she wished to go back. The superintendent said she could go if she liked, but she would not pay her passage home. This quite upset Mrs. ——'s calculations, as she had reckoned upon a free passage to England.

She became very insolent indeed, and was obliged to be reminded that, if she did not submit to the rules of the house, we were in a military hospital and could call in the assistance of the authorities. The vision of "arrest" rather frightened her, she contented herself with warning us what we might expect when she did get back to England—she would expose all our doings.

One of the nurses came to report her threats in great terror.

"Oh, if you please, ma'am, she does say such dreadful things that she is a-going to do. We shall be as good as *massacreed* when she gets home!"

"Well, never mind," we said, "let her *only* go away and get home, and we will see when the massacre comes."

She left the house on the day the vessel for England was to sail, went to the British Consul, and I believe prevailed upon him to give her a passage to Malta. He probably did not want her among the British subjects at Constantinople. The other discharged nurse was sent to Galata to embark for England, but contrived to get away from the person in charge and ran into Constantinople. We never could trace her afterwards. Such was the consequence of sending out women of inferior character to such a work of trial and temptation. We felt it bitterly when we wished so much that a good example should be set to the men, and that we should raise and influence them for the better; it would have been all undone by these women, while to them, poor creatures, a military hospital was the very worst place that could be imagined rife with every sort of temptation.

A few weeks only had elapsed since the departure of the two women I have mentioned, when disgraceful misconduct caused the dismissal of a third. Ere a passage could be had for her another was obliged to go, from her habits of intoxication, and she had been one most highly recommended; and to hear her talk you would think she was a very religious person. These two left together. The chaplain himself offered to see them on board, and his task was no light one, for during the whole *caique* voyage down the Bosphorus every sort of abuse and bad language were showered down upon his head.

Our trials were not ended. A similar case of bad conduct obliged the dismissal of one whom we had looked upon as one of our best nurses. Another was found intoxicated in the wards; these two went a few weeks or two more for the same reason; and so, on till, out of the twenty-one, in less than eight months we had eleven left. To our profound astonishment we found that our sending home so many gave great umbrage to the authorities at home. They thought fit to send a reproof, demanding more particulars of the cases, and evidently displeased at the number sent back.

They were respectfully reminded that our superintendent's duties did not include the reformation of women of loose character and immoral habits, nor did we imagine the authorities would require details which were often too terrible to dwell on. We certainly did expect that the ladies intrusted with the arduous charge of controlling the nurses in our Eastern hospitals were better judges of what class of persons were or were not fit for that work, than those who, safe in English homes, had perhaps never entered an hospital ward at all—certainly never toiled in a military one night and day.

Of the remaining nine two were very unsatisfactory (Mrs. Woodward, who came from Oxford, and had been recommended by Dr. Acland, was quite an exception to what has been said. She was perfectly respectable and trustworthy, and altogether a most valuable person). The other six were respectable and industrious, and under a lady's supervision did very well, but not a single one, except Mrs. Woodward, could be trusted alone. They would give things to favourite patients without the surgeon's leave, or omit to carry out his orders unless they were made to do it.

In ordinary hospitals the nurses constantly do this. I have been told by medical men that, humanly speaking, they have known lives among their patients lost by the nurses' disobedience; but in English hospitals the doctors submit to this—they must have nurses, they can get no better—while in Eastern hospitals the nursing was acknowledged to be an experiment, and it was of the greatest importance strict obedience should be paid to the commands of the surgeons, or we knew not but that it might end in their refusing to accept our aid altogether. It was no easy thing to introduce a new element into the beaten routine of military hospitals, and needed great care, skill, and prudence in those intrusted with its management to do it successfully.

CHAPTER 17

Cooks Sent Out by Government

I will now speak more fully of what I can with justice say was the most important part of our work. When Miss Stanley first entered Koulali Hospital and asked the principal medical officer what sort of work her nurses should undertake, the answer at once was that they should undertake the cooking and seeing the diets given at proper times.

"It is not the surgical cases," said one of the first-class staff-surgeons, "for which we require your assistance. Their wounds are as well or better dressed by the regular dressers, but it is the medical cases which require watching and feeding, and just that constant care which nurses can and we cannot give, and a large proportion of the present cases require good nursing more than medical skill."

We have described the first formation of the kitchen, its gradual advance from charcoal brasiers to a shed in the yard, and a kitchen in the *Sultan's* quarters of the hospital. This latter we gave up when we left our apartments there, as it was required for the officers' use. The shed in the barrack-yard was enlarged and improved, and all the extra cooking carried on. there, but still it was far from possessing all necessary conveniences.

At the General Hospital for all these months the Sisters' extra diet cooking had been done on brasiers; they had no storeroom, and were obliged to keep their free gifts in their own apartments. In the Barrack Hospital we had a good-size storeroom, but sadly wanting shelves and other improvements; and there was one great hindrance which stood in the way of real improvement in this department: the materials for the extra diets were drawn daily from the purveyor's store by the orderlies of each ward, according to them diet roll, and then brought to the kitchen to be cooked.

Great waste was the natural consequence of this. Small quantities of sago, rice, arrowroot, were being cooked for each separate ward, while, if all were done at once, half the quantity would be sufficient; and, as I have before mentioned, for any mistake in drawing the rations, or for any deficiency in the food, there was no remedy except through private gifts, which were quite inadequate to the claims thus made upon them.

When the purveyor-in-chief visited Koulali this difficulty was laid before him, and he remedied it at once by giving the lady in charge of the store-room authority to draw on the stores and use the materials according to her own judgment. Finding that the General Hospital stood greatly in want of a kitchen and store-room, he furnished them; two small rooms in the building fronting the quadrangle were chosen for this purpose, and the Reverend Mother, assisted by Sister M——J——, undertook the management.

It was all that was wanting to make the General Hospital perfect. The two rooms were beautifully fitted up—the kitchen with oven and boilers, and brasiers built into the wall where frying and boiling could go on—the store room furnished with shelves and drawers; and when these arrangements were completed the kitchen was well supplied with cooking utensils, plates, and dishes, and, what we admired most of all, small round tins, with a coyer attached to it by a chain—these were for the dinners to be served in, and thus kept hot in their travels from the kitchen to the wards.

The store-room was filled with every comfort that could be wished for. Preserved soups of all kinds—we had never been able till now to draw these from the stores—we had in the winter a large quantity of them sent out by Mr. Gamble to Miss Nightingale at Scutari, and she sent on a part to Koulali. They were much prized by the men and also by the then overworked nurses, who at that time were very thankful for anything that enabled them to procure a diet quickly, and Mr. Gamble's preserved meat only requires to be heated and hot water added and it is most excellent soup ready at hand.

"It's the beautifullest thing I ever tasted," said one patient. "That's the stuff to do us good," remarked many others.

Now the store-room shelves had plenty of this soup, and plenty of essence of beef (an invaluable thing in sickness), sago and arrowroot, rice, sugar, gelatine in large quantities, wine and brandy, soda-water, eggs, lemons and oranges; other comforts were afterwards added. The diets were in a very different state; the fowls and chops did not look like the same, and the men said they tasted quite different. Rice-puddings were an important branch in the extra-diet kitchen. It was difficult to make them well, owing to the inferior kind of milk, rice, and eggs. The Reverend Mother solved the problem, and as good rice puddings as anyone could desire were sent out and gave great satisfaction.

We found it, however, quite impossible to make the puddings properly without using more materials than were allowed us by the diet roll, so that we used our privilege of drawing on the stores to make up the deficiency. For all the expenditure of the store-room an account was required to be kept and sent in to the purveyor's.

Sister M—— ——J was an excellent accountant. It was a pleasure to look at her books, and they gained great commendation when they went in to the purveyor's office to be checked. At the Barrack Hospital improvements in the extra diets went on, the kitchen was enlarged and furnished with fireplaces, additional ovens, &c.

The rice-pudding reform was introduced; after we saw the beautiful ones sent out by the Sisters, we were ambitious ours should be as good, and the superintendent and the lady in charge of the kitchen begged the Reverend Mother to give them lessons in this branch of cooking, which she kindly did; so they went up to the General Hospital and saw how they were made, and watched the general routine of the kitchen, and then tried to copy it below—for the Sisters' long experience in all matters concerning the care of the poor and sick gave them a great superiority over us, and they were ever ready to show us their method and to enter into our difficulties, and these, in our extra-diet kitchen in Turkey, were not a few. Milk that would turn, eggs the half or more than half the number rotten, the rice filled with dirt, are great obstacles in the construction of puddings, so also are green lemons when you want to make lemonade.

Most of these articles were supplied to the hospital by contract, and when it was a little more difficult than usual to get things—such as milk in the hot weather, or lemons when the season for them was past—they used to send *anything* they could get hold of, and the purveyor would have kept them had we not had permission from the purveyor-in-chief to send back inferior articles, for he said the contractors were well paid by Government, and ought and should send articles fit for use.

We soon had excellent rice and rather better milk, but it was impossible to get really good milk anywhere. Lady Stratford de Redcliffe used to send some milk daily to the "Home," from Therapia, which was the best that could be had, and by heating this directly it came in we prevented it from turning, but if this precaution was neglected in the middle of the day it became sour. Good eggs we tried hard for, but could not procure, and were obliged to be content with breaking dozens of rotten ones to arrive at the good. The green lemons we returned, and after some battles with the contractors we got others.

Gelatine was the next difficulty. There was a call for jelly: of course, no calves' feet could be had, so we tried gelatine, one kind of which made it nicely, while the other made it so very thick and bad we could not send it into the wards. It was by no means sufficient just to state this to the purveyor and ask for it to be changed, he thought it would "do very well," so we had to be very resolute to get our way.

The Barrack Hospital extra-diet kitchen had a cook who was a civilian (a good many of whom had been sent out by government). This was a great improvement, as it is difficult to find cooks among the soldiers, and when they are found and practised, they are liable—as the orderlies—to be ordered up to their regiment. At the General Hospital, however, Sister M—— J—— had a soldier for a cook who gave her great satisfaction.

The routine of the extra store-rooms was as follows: They were opened at nine in the morning; the nurse who assisted the lady, or Sister, sweeping and dusting, while the lady looked over the total abstract and ladies' requisitions. The former was made by the purveyor's clerk, who examined the die-rolls of each ward and then made an abstract of the extra diets required of them, and sent it in to the lady or Sister; the latter were for such articles as the ladies required extra to the diet rolls, such as they had verbal permission to give, and for such articles as they wished to keep in their cupboards for emergencies. They were like the following:—

(No. 50.)   July 19, 1855
Required for 3 Lower Ward, Koulali Hospital 4 quarts lemon-

ade; 3 *do.* milk; 4 *do.* arrowroot; 2 doz. eggs; jelly for two; ½lb. of butter; 2 doz. biscuits.

  Miss ——— (Signed) Sister M—— A——.

 Every lady and Sister sent in a requisition. Except in a case of great emergency they were only permitted to send once a day for all they wanted throughout it, as otherwise irregularity was caused. These requisitions were then served; the articles for each ward were arranged in order, in addition to the requirements of the diet rolls. Then the bell was rung and in an instant a group of orderlies rushed across the barrack-yard to see who would be in time first and carry off his extras. Requisitions from the medical officers came in at all hours, and were instantly attended to.

 At 12.30 the bell again rang, and the orderlies assembled to fetch their dinners; for this purpose they had wooden trays, on which were counted out the number of fowls, chops, potatoes, each required, then they returned again for rice pudding, macaroni pudding, pints of rice or sago milk; in a quarter of an hour all were served; then came diets of sick officers, for among the large body attached to the hospitals there were generally one or two on the sick list. At two the store room was closed till four; at five the bell summoned the orderlies to fetch the night drinks—lemonade, barley-water, or tea, as were ordered; arrowroot or beef-tea was again made if required.

 In the evening the lady in charge wrote her requisitions on the purveyor's stores for such articles as she would require for her store room the next day. On Sundays the hours were slightly altered, owing to the arrangement that all persons in the store room and kitchen should attend Divine service; but though each had the opportunity afforded them, the patients were in no ways neglected.

 Most amusing scenes went on at times in the extra-diet kitchen. The orderlies did not like the civilian cook, and he returned the compliment; they were perpetually telling tales of each other. Once when Miss ——— was detained from her work for a few days by illness, she received the following note from the cook:—

> Madam—I wish to acquaint you about the malice that is existing among some of the orderlies towards me, and the other servants in the kitchen. I believe the cause to be not having a free intercourse in the kitchen as formerly, and moreover, an antipathy towards me for doing my duty. If I have not done my duty to the best of my ability, I will refer to your honourable

decision. Yesterday evening I had a requisition for six pints of chocolate at 7 p.m., when I was at my room; I was in the act of dressing when the orderly came, I made haste over to the kitchen and the ladies' store was locked, therefore, I could not comply with the requisition. This morning he made a special report to the doctor. Under these circumstances, and with your kind permission, I would like for my welfare and also for the best mode of regulating the kitchen, to have some restrictions. Regarding this, I hope, madam, with my greatest respect, that you will take interest in these few lines. I remain, madam,
  Your humble servant.

T. R., Cook

 There were a good many Greeks also employed in the kitchen (for the labour of fetching water from the extreme end of the barrack-yard required a good many hands, and chopping wood was another piece of heavy work); the Greeks were a great torment, they were perpetually running off, staying away for a day or so and then coming back, and quarrelling and fighting among themselves, and being idle and disobedient. One had to send messages almost every day to the sergeant in charge of the Greeks, "Wanted a Greek."

 At last came an Italian named Constantine, he was an old man but worth six Greeks. Always at hand, willing, gentle, and obedient, he picked up a few sentences of English very fast and was very proud of his acquirements. His favourite employment was to help the lady putting out the stores, lifting the heavy weights for her and so on; he was quite honest, but he and cook could not agree and there were dreadful battles.

 Cook complained so of his disobedience in the kitchen that Miss —— was forced to speak to him, and it was very absurd, as she could not speak either Greek or Italian, and had to express her displeasure by using the little English Constantine knew and by signs. Constantine understood quite well, and made a vehement defence; he danced about the room, and, with many gesticulations, gave her to understand that *"Monsieur Cook"* was so unreasonable, he wanted Constantine to be in the kitchen when he was helping *madame* in the store room, and that he could not be in two places at once, and *Monsieur Cook* was so rough he called out so loud and was not quiet like *madame*. However, the reproof did good, and the kitchen was more peaceable.

 Monsieur Soyer paid a visit to Koulali before the improvements in the extra-diet kitchen had taken place. He offered to show a better way of making the hospital tea, *i.e.*, that issued from the large general kitchen for all the diets. There was room for improvement, for it was the most wretched stuff possible. Monsieur Soyer's was much better, and yet he made it, he said, with exactly the same proportions as before. I do not think his improvements were attended to at the kitchen, but as it did not come within our province I cannot be sure.

Monsieur Soyer made his tea in the little kitchen outside the Convalescent Hospital. The medical officers and the ladies came to taste it, and it was an amusing scene: the group outside tasting the tea, the tiny kitchen, which just held Monsieur Soyer and his assistants, and the patients of the Convalescent Hospital looking on and wondering what was going to happen to their tea that night.

CHAPTER 18

Affection of the Irish Soldiers for Their Nuns

The routine of the hospital was often interrupted by the arrival of sick, who came in numbers varying from 50 to 100. We seldom had more than a few hours' notice, and often not that. Sometimes it was not till the steamer was alongside the quay that we knew they were coming; this arose from all the sick from the camp being sent to Scutari first and the steamer coming back from thence to Koulali.

When they arrived, there was a general commotion; the principal medical officer, the *commandant*, and most of the medical staff went down to the quay to receive them and see them carefully carried up. Orderlies ran hither and thither, ward-masters and nurses were in a bustle getting beds prepared. The kitchen staff was hard at work to get coppers full of hot water, and fires lighted in readiness for the doctor's orders. Ladies and Sisters looking after the clean linen.

A different scene it was truly from that which used to be presented a few months back, when the poor sufferers came in and no beds were ready and no clean linen, and no nurses to attend and watch by them. A blessed change indeed it was.

There was a division made of the sick, part going to the Barrack and part going to the General hospitals. All who were able walked, the rest were borne on stretchers. As soon as the sick were in their beds, requisitions began to pour in. One ward ordered beef tea, another negus, a third *good* tea. The orderly officer for the day was in great request as he must sign the requisitions, or give the Sisters and ladies verbal orders from which they might write their own requisitions.

Very touching incidents often occurred among the sick just come in; they were so astonished to find so many comforts ready, and so many hands to minister to them. The quantity of clean linen was a great wonderment; they said they had more here in a week than in the camp for months together.

The poor Irish soldiers were much charmed at the sight of the nuns—"Our own Sisters," they would fondly say.

I remember one poor man brought in who was a Roman Catholic; he was so ill he could not speak, could neither ask for temporal comfort or spiritual consolation, but he looked up into the face of the Sister who was attending on him, and perceiving the crucifix hanging from her girdle eagerly seized it with his dying grasp and pressed it fervently to his lips.

The national spirit of the Irish was very strong; it was pleasing to see their reverence and affection for their priests and the nuns. The Irish orderlies used to be delighted beyond measure to be allowed to wait on the Catholic chaplain; nothing was so great a treat as to be doing something for "his riverence."

There were amusing scenes sometimes with Irish sailors. There was a wharf just below Koulali, where steamers often came to coal; once or twice the crews were principally Irish. The sailors had leave to go on shore, and dispersed themselves about the country; they went through the hospital wards, evidently delighted at the comfortable appearance of the men. They looked at and admired everything; but when they met their countrywomen—the Sisters of Mercy—in the barrack-yard they were quite overjoyed.

When they found that they lived at the General Hospital they poured up the hill in troops to visit them and attend their chapel. Many who had not attended to their religious duties for years were persuaded to do so now. They did not forget the ladies either, but were overheard one night on the quay to be talking the matter over, and saying, *however* those ladies could have come out all this way with nobody to take care of them was past *their* conception.

Butter was a great treat to our men; before the arrival of the new purveyor-in-chief the bread was so dry and sour that it was difficult even for those in health to force it down unless very hungry. No butter was at that time given on the diet roll. We asked the leave of the medical officers to give it to our patients. This was granted, and we were enabled to obtain it through the kindness of friends in England, who sent us money for this and such-like purposes. It will gratify them to know that many and many a poor fellow had a comfortable meal through their consideration.

We are glad to take this opportunity of thanking them for the warm, affectionate sympathy and ready help they so often afforded us, not only in sending us money and other presents but for the personal trouble they took in the matter. We had but to write to England and say we wanted such and such a thing and it was sent by the first opportunity, and not only this but we often received letters begging us to write and say what things would be useful. Little schoolchildren sent us money—small sums they had saved, and wished to be sent to the "ladies who nursed the sick soldiers."

Could these friends have seen the glistening eyes with which the poor men listened to the account of their kindness, and have heard their hearty "God bless them—God bless them !" they would have been more than rewarded. It would have pleased them to have gone round our wards with us at tea-time, accompanied by our butter-bowl, and have seen the grateful look of each patient as he received his small portion, and have heard his exclamation, "Why, here's actually a bit of butter—that *is* nice and homelike!"

Many would keep half their portions till next morning's breakfast. It certainly was very unlike English butter, and we sometimes wondered how they could eat it with such evident enjoyment; but long months of hardship and almost starvation had taught them to be easily satisfied with what many in England would have grumbled at. Our means of procuring them this comfort of course soon came to an end. It was not fair to give butter in one ward and not in another, and one £3 after another was quickly spent in providing a whole hospital with butter, even once or twice a week, as it cost from 3s. to 4s. a pound. 4s. we always paid for it when we bought it at the canteens, but we could procure it at 3s. if we bought casks of £2 or £3 value at Constantinople.

When Mr. Robertson came he ordered butter to be had in the stores, and we drew it upon requisition, and gave it when we thought the men really needed it. Next, we happened to be complaining to one of the officer's wives of the sour bread furnished to the hospital, which also came to our own table. She said it was very strange, their bread was beautiful, as good or better than English. We found this arose from the officers' rations being drawn from the commissariat department, while ours came, like the patients', from the purveying, and that these two departments had separate contractors for bread.

Upon this being represented to the purveyor-in-chief he changed the bread contract at Midsummer, and from that time the hospital was supplied with excellent bread, the contractor being Mr. Hamelin, the Armenian Minister at Bebek. From his bakery long previous to this we procured biscuits which were very good. They were twelve *piastres* the *ock* (an *ock* is about two and a half pounds), so that they are much cheaper as well as better than any we could have procured in the French shops at Pera.

We spent a good deal of our free-gift money in purchasing them, for we often found men who were very weak could eat biscuits when they could not swallow or digest bread. Eventually biscuits, like every other imaginable comfort, could be freely drawn from Government stores.

The bad washing, and consequent deficiency in the linen department, had been severely felt from the first, but there was no remedy. At Scutari the washing we heard, was now well regulated, being done on the spot by means of washing machines, but this could not be done at Koulali, as there was no building which could be made into a washhouse; all that could be done was to place the linen stores under the charge of the Sisters and ladies.

It was a point on which Mr. Robertson was very anxious. He had rooms fitted up for this purpose at both hospitals; at the upper one it was under the charge of Sister J—— M——, who began hers first, and it was conducted in beautiful order.

The linen stores of the Lower Hospital was under Miss ——, and nurses assisted in both stores.

The care of the linen stores was a very laborious work. The lady superintendent, in addition to her numerous duties, spent much of her time in those at the Barrack Hospital; she kept the accounts, and brought it by degrees into perfect shape and order.

The washing was sent across to Bebek, where it was contracted for by the Protestant Armenian Minister there. It was executed by Greeks, who sometimes thought fit to work and sometimes not, so that often the washing was in arrear. A great quantity of linen always had to be returned to be washed again a momentary dip in the water evidently having been the extent of labour bestowed upon it.

When the washing came over it was taken to the sergeants, who had charge of the soiled linen (this department being of course under sergeant and orderlies), clean linen was then sent to the linen stores upon requisition. The ladies and Sisters who worked at the linen stores spent their whole daytime there, only leaving it for meals and evening recreations. Twice a-week they received the clean linen, and after sending back the badly washed they proceeded to sort the articles, then followed the folding, and lastly the mending.

Twice a-week the ladies and Sisters of the respective wards sent in their requisitions, the ladies at the linen store served these, put the different articles in bundles for the wards, and then the orderlies fetched them. The Sisters and ladies had in their wards, linen cupboards (under lock and key), where they kept a small quantity of linen ready in case of sudden illness or fresh cases coming in.

It took a long time before the linen stores were arranged in a satisfactory manner, but we at length succeeded, and had now the pleasure of knowing that there was no comfort required in sickness which was not supplied to the British soldier. He had the best medical skill and suitable attention, food as good as could be had in Turkey, and linen in as great a quantity as in the hospitals at home. The work in the linen stores was so very arduous that the other ladies, when their work in the wards was lighter than usual, often dropped in to lend their assistance towards reducing the interminable mending.

CHAPTER 19

The Free Gift Store

The Free Gift Store has often been referred to; it was the store supplied by the gifts of the people of England, who generously and promptly sent them out to their suffering army; and although much disappointment has, I know, been experienced by many on hearing that numbers of these packages never reached their destination, yet it will be a satisfaction to many to learn the benefit given by that portion which did arrive.

The free gifts had to be carefully sorted, for often a good many useless things were sent out. Some portion of the free gifts sent to Scutari was forwarded to Koulali. Others were sent straight to us, and some we purchased with money sent out from England. Small-tooth combs we bought in great numbers when the hospital was crowded, for they were much needed. An old Turk used to sit at the hospital gate with a stall of trifles, and had some small-tooth combs—he looked so surprised when we broke his stall of them.

At first, we had no separate store to keep our free gifts in, but they were kept in one of the government stores, and under charge of the sergeant who had charge of the first. He was an amusing individual, very unlike the soldiers in general, and so very grand that he thought it rather a condescension on his part to attend to us. After a time, a shed in the barrack yard, that had been a canteen, was given up to our use, and was by the engineer officer made into a nice little building in three compartments:—First, the superintendent's room; second, the Free Gift Store; third, for packing cases, &c. As soon as we could carry our free gifts into this store, the superintendent arranged them all in order on the shelves, with which the room was furnished.

Sometimes it looked quite full, but never remained so for long together; a party of invalids ordered home soon made a hole in it. This store was under the Lady superintendent's charge. She saw the things unpacked and arranged, and received the requisitions signed by the ladies and Sisters for what they considered their men needed before going to England or to the camp.

When Miss Stanley was lady superintendent she divided the gifts among the ladies in charge of the wards, who distributed them according to their own judgment, and this plan was followed out after Miss Stanley's departure. The unpacking of the boxes was often quite affecting. Many a wish was expressed that the kind contributors could see the pleasure their gifts gave. There were packages of lint, of mittens, of comforters made up and enclosed as the gift of the poor. There was one packet of sugar-candy, with a note in a large round hand, "For the sick soldiers, from a little girl." Another "from a little German girl." Quantities of pocket handkerchiefs were also sent; flannels, Jerseys, socks, nightcaps; some crimson pocket handkerchiefs gave great delight, cotton shirts were also valued.

We found the free gifts principally useful as affording us the means of giving necessaries to the men going to England, for they would otherwise have taken that voyage often without a change of linen or any warm clothing. The men who came down in the winter and spring had usually lost their kits in the camp, and so were quite destitute. Long afterwards, when the men did bring their kits down with them, we always enquired what was deficient in them.

After the quarter-master had given what he thought requisite, we then gave them articles from our store; so that it was always busy work when the men were going home, for another rule was not to give the things till just as they were going away, that there might be no temptation thrown in their way to sell their clothes for drink. Consequently, all had to be done in a few hours. The ladies wrote their list of what the men wanted, and the superintendent gave them out, and as soon as we had given them, they went on board.

The scene at these times was always very interesting. Groups of poor fellows in each ward just risen from their beds and dressed in the uniform of the different regiments, packing up their kits, and reiterating their thanks for the clothes they had just received. Orderlies running about trying to get the invalids' dinners a little sooner than the usual hour, that the invalids might have a good meal before starting. Comrades who had fought together on the field of battle, or suffered side by side in the trenches before Sebastopol, wishing each other goodbye, those who were left behind sending messages to them friends in England.

Chaplains giving away Bibles and prayer books, and as a last kind thought very often finding a quantity of tobacco for them to smoke on the voyage. Sisters and ladies having a last word with those whom they had long tended, and whom in all human probability they would never meet again in this world, many of these with tears in their eyes loading them with blessings, and earnestly promising (what they well knew would more than compensate for any trouble they might have taken) that they would be different men henceforth to what they had been before they came into the hospital.

And now the order is loudly given at the entrance of each ward, "The invalids for England to proceed to the shore," and they slowly depart—orderlies carrying the kits of those who are too weak to do so themselves, and some of the wounded and incurable being taken down on stretchers. They all pass down the barrack yard and through the main guard entrance, which is crowded with doctors and officers. One of these accompanies the invalids as far as Scutari, where they embark in a larger vessel for England—and now the little steamer is ready—the poor fellows are all on board, and we watch them depart with a silent prayer for their safe arrival in old England.

On Mondays and Thursdays, patients were discharged from the convalescent hospital to proceed to Scutari, from thence to go to the camp, and what we considered deficient in their kits were made up from the Free Gift Store, so that it had enough to do to supply all these demands. Sometimes it did get alarmingly low, but somehow, by hook or by crook, it got up again, and we always bad enough to give. The men were so grateful for these gifts, and so pleased with them. An amusing letter was sent to one of us once which I insert—the cotton shirts the writer speaks of had been given but not the rest of the free gifts, and he was very much afraid none were coming.

Miss —— Please if in your power to let me have the following articles, *viz.*, one pair of slippers, for my feet are very sore; one red scarf; one nightcap; one pocket-handkerchief.

N.B.—None of the above have I received, though you have supplied me well with clean linen for the voyage, for which I sincerely thank you, and your kindness to me and to everyone in the ward shall never be forgotten or neglected in the prayers of your humble servant,

Corporal G——

A flannel shirt and a pair of drawers would be most welcome indeed, for I have one of each, and I'd like to have a change.

G——

Occasionally soldiers' wives would be leaving with the invalids. There were, however, very few of these women at Koulali; the greater number of them were at Scutari, where they received much kindness and assistance from Lady Alicia Blackwood when they left for England, if they were deserving cases. They also received clothes for the voyage. She commissioned Sister Anne to undertake the business for her at Koulali. They were often in great distress for clothes, both for themselves and children, and clothes were far more valuable to them than money, owing to the great difficulty of procuring and high price to be given for them in Pera. Lady Napier was also very kind in sending clothes to Sister Anne to distribute among them.

One poor woman, who washed for the officers, had fallen asleep late one night in the wash-house, and her clothes caught fire. She was frightfully burnt, and was carried to a room over one of the wards where doctors and nurses attended to her. For eight or nine months she lay there unable to move, her husband also in the hospital. They were both invalided home, but she was not able to undertake the voyage, and when we left Koulali she was still there.

Chapter 20

A Fearful Accident

There are several pretty walks around Koulali, but we did not often take them as we were afraid to be far out of call of the sentries; our usual walks were to the Turkish cemetery, or the *Sultan's* kiosk.

The cemetery was on a hill a little beyond the General Hospital; it is a grove of cypresses interspersed with white marble tombstones. The immense extent of these cemeteries custom of planting a cypress at each grave. This custom is not now so general, the Turks never place more than one body in a grave.

The Turkish name for Koulali is *Kulleh Baglidshessi*, or the garden of the tower. There is a legend attached to it. Sultan Selim the 1st was so enraged against his son Suleikam that he commanded his *vizier* to have him strangled. The *vizier*, however, risked his own life to save that of the prince. He confined him for three years in a tower at Koulali. Selim one day repented himself of his cruelty—for he had no other children and then the *vizier* thought fit to confess his disobedience. Selim was succeeded by Suleiman, who pulled down the tower and planted a beautiful garden and fountain on the spot of his captivity.

The *Sultan's* kiosk is built on the point of the highest hill above Koulali. It was such labour to climb it that we seldom went, but when we did gain the summit, the view was magnificent, for we could see miles of the Bosphorus and the Sea of Marmora.

The next village to Koulali is Candilee, and it is a lovely spot; its ancient name meant stream-girt, from the strength of the current which washes its banks, but now it is called Candilee, *i.e.*, hung with lanterns. It is impossible to describe the exquisite beauty of the views from Candilee. Several English gentlemen have country houses here; from one we visited we saw plainly the Black Sea, the Sea of Marmora, almost the whole extent of the Bosphorus, hills, and palaces, and groves without number—Europe and Asia at one glance. The advantage of living on the summit of these hills is their extreme coolness—the only drawback being the labour of ascending them.

Opposite Candilee, on the European coast, is the village of Bebek, with its lovely bay, a favourite resort of Europeans. Here are several American families, and also French and German. Here are also two colleges—one a French Catholic, under the order of Lazarist Fathers, the other a Protestant Armenian, under the care of an Armenian gentleman. There is also a small convent and *enfants trouvés*, belonging to the *Soeurs de la Charité*. We visited these three institutions; the first contained about 500 boys, who were all dressed like French soldiers, and among their other studies military exercises are diligently learned, a French soldier being their instructor. Boys of every nation are there—Turks even send their sons, so that the facility of acquiring languages is very great. We counted ten that are spoken in the house.

We were most courteously received by the Superior, and conducted over the college. We saw the library and the laboratory, and the boys at their gymnastics, and heard their singing in the little chapel. The music was an improvement on the general character of French music in the East, but the chapel was so much too small for the large body of voice accompanied by an organ, that we could hardly judge of its merits. We enquired whether the Turkish boys attend the chapel. The answer was "seldom." It was entirely voluntary; if they wished for religious instruction they had it, but they were not forced to hear it.

The superior himself conducted us to the *Maison de Saint Joseph* close by, belonging to the Sisters of Charity; they are sent from the convent at Galata. Their house is for sick children and the *enfants trouvés*, on a very small scale, however, in comparison to the well-known institutions of Paris.

Here again the amalgamation of different nations struck us—a *Soeur* was standing at a window holding in her arms a dark-eyed Italian baby, a fair-haired German child was climbing up her knee, while a little sickly-looking Russian sat beside her. Groups of other little ones, some suffering from sickness and others the lonely and forsaken, played about the room. Four Sisters were in charge of them, gathering, as these sweet Sisters ever do the most desolate and afflicted of God's creatures into their loving care. The college and Sister's house stand in a lovely situation, half-way up the hill, looking down on the Bosphorus.

We visited the Protestant Armenian College, and were most kindly received by the principal and his family. We were conducted over the college library, dormitories, &c., but it being the recess we did not see the pupils. The college is intended for young Armenian men belonging to the sect of Protestant Armenians. Mr. H———, the principal, kindly invited us to spend an evening with his family, and walk to see the French camp, then lying about a mile from their residence— the sight, he said, was worth looking at.

We accepted the invitation, and afterwards spent a pleasant evening at Bebek, but in the interim cholera had broken out in the French camp, which had been moved elsewhere; we returned home that evening by moonlight and the Bosphorus looked like a plain of silver light. Clearly in the brilliance stood out the hills and surrounding houses; now and then a *caique* darted past us like a bird, so swiftly did it go; in the distance was the city, looking dim and shadowy; the current was with us and our row took us only ten minutes, when against the current we were half an hour or more coming across.

About this time, we had occasion to visit Therapia, and some of us who had there spent the first six weeks of our lives in the East were desirous of seeing it in its summer aspect; on our journey up the Bosphorus we passed the village of Yenikoi, which was full of huts containing the sick of the Sardinian Army. A great many Greeks live at Yenikoi, for here begins the part of the river where the Christians are allowed to build country houses.

When we reached Therapia a change was indeed apparent. The *Sultan's* palace was converted into a convalescent hospital for the British, and was in beautiful order. We walked in the extensive grounds, under the shade of the magnificent trees which must form such a delightful walk for the invalids.

After visiting our kind friends at the hospital, we walked through the town along the quay to the embassy gardens—they were indeed lovely—the lilac Judas trees and acacia in full blossom, large white arums geraniums and myrtles grew in profusion, while the garden of Lord Napier's house was a wilderness of China roses. We climbed the steep path up to the flag-staff and gazed on the once familiar view so very lovely now in the summer brightness.

The sweet waters of Asia are situated just below Anatoli Hissar, and thus exactly opposite to Humeli Hissar; these two fortresses are called by Europeans the Castles of Europe and Asia, being built as defences for the narrowest part of the Bosphorus. Here Darius crossed with his army, with horses, elephants, and camels, on his expedition against the Scythians.

On a stone pillar on each shore were inscribed the names of the nations who crossed with him. Here was also the rock cut into the form of a throne, where Darius sat and contemplated the march of his army from Asia to Europe; to the building of the walls of this fortress were applied the pillars and altars of the Church of St. Michael which had been built at Koulali. The Castle of Europe was built 1451, two years before the Ottoman conquest of Constantinople; the Castle of Asia had been erected some time previously.

This latter was once called Guzel Hissar, *i.e.*, the beautiful castle; but terrible tales would be told could those ruined walls find a tongue, for afterwards they named the beautiful castle the Black Tower, for many hundreds here met their death from torture and cruelty. Strange that in a spot which God has made fair beyond the power of language to describe, man has delighted in the cry of agony. Many other armies have followed the example of Darius, and crossed the Bosphorus at this point—Persians, Goths, Latins, and Turks.

The Castle of Asia is entirely in ruins, but the Castle of Europe is still standing. It was built intending to form the Turkish characters of M H M D, which make the name of the founder Mahomet II.

After rowing three miles down we came to the narrow creek leading to the sweet waters, about a quarter of a mile in length the name of this creek or small river is Göhsu, *i.e*., the heavenly water. It is considered the most lovely spot in Asia—the water has rather a sweet taste, from whence has arisen its name—it is always called sweet waters. Each side is hung with trees bending down to the water's edge. At the end of the creek, we generally landed and walked in the green fields beyond. The pleasure of this excursion principally consisted in our being able to say, we could fancy ourselves in England. The scenery rather reminded some of us of that in the south of Devonshire.

On Friday (the Turkish Sabbath), the valley of the sweet waters is the favourite rendezvous of the Turkish ladies. They assemble beneath some large green trees in a field on the banks of the sweet waters; close by rises a new palace the *Sultan* is building. The windings of the Bosphorus, and its hills crowned with kiosks, and its banks crowded with houses can be seen for some distance as one stands in the valley of sweet waters. The white and ivy-covered towers of the Castle of Europe form a striking picture in the landscape; near the banks is a marble fountain, richly ornamented with carving; but on a Friday the scene in the valley itself almost distracted one's attention from the landscape.

Under the trees are spread carpets and cushions of various colours, upon these recline the Turkish ladies sitting in groups clothed in dresses of every bright hue—green, blue, red, pink, yellow, orange, violet, &c. Some are smoking, some are drinking coffee out of their tiny cups, some buying sweatmeats and toys—vendors of these are straying about in all directions—children in their quaint Turkish dresses, miniatures of their elders, are playing about—heavy Turkish carriages containing the *sultanas* and other ladies of high rank, drive slowly round the field—Greek ladies and gentlemen, and children, and French *ditto*. Here and there an Albanian diversifies the scene.

We here observed one of the most beautiful women we had seen since we came to Turkey. She was seated on a pile of cushions under a large tree, and was dressed in a pale lavender cashmere, a white *yashmac, feridjee*, and yellow gloves—these latter articles being only worn by ladies of high rank; and from the number of slaves which surrounded her we guessed her to be a person of distinction.

It was her perfect grace of attitude which struck us; for although one may often see a beautiful face in Turkey, it is generally accompanied by an awkward, ungraceful carriage. But like a heroine of some old Eastern tale sat the lady of whom we speak. How we longed for an artist's pencil to draw her picture, and the panorama around. Could it be real, or were we looking through a kaleidoscope?

As it grew dark the ladies entered their carriages or *caiques* to return home, and we too sought ours, and were soon at home, for the current bore us swiftly along.

The currents of the Bosphorus are very strong, and on some days, without visible reason, will be much more so than on others. Immediately before our house was one of the strongest; it often drove quite a large ship back—indeed the larger ships and vessels seemed more under its influence than the small boats; for they, after two or three vain attempts to stem it, would go cautiously into the middle of the stream, and so avoid some of its fury.

But the ships were helpless without the aid of a steamer; they turned round and round, and we often expected to see the yards come through our windows. In fact, it once happened that a ship did injure one of the rooms, and another knocked down part of our garden wall.

On one occasion, too, we witnessed from our windows a sad accident. A poor man, owing to a concussion between two boats, fell into the seething waters, his rescue was impossible, and he was drowned before our eyes. This current is called *sheitan akindisi*, or devil's current, and to it there belongs a legend. A *sultana* in her *caique* was once proceeding down the Bosphorus when she met a number of persons going to worship in a Christian church, upon which she ordered the church to be pulled down. On her return her *caique* was seized by the current and upset, but all the attendants and boatmen were saved, the *sultana* only was lost. Almost every spot in Turkey has some old legend attached to it.

One of our favourite expeditions was to the lovely gardens of Bebek. They belonged to the *Sultan's* chief physician, who very kindly threw them open to the English or French. It was refreshing after a long hot day's work in the hospital, to row across and wander among the orange and citron groves and sit under the shadowy trees, while the air around was laden with the sweet scent of innumerable flowers, the birds singing over our heads the only sound, and everything above, beneath, and around bright with beauty. We could have fancied ourselves in fairyland—"*And the fire-flies glance in the myrtle boughs,*"—

completed the dream-like loveliness of the whole scene. The gardens are most beautifully laid out, terrace above terrace, and bower succeeding bower, and many a winding path, forming gradual ascents to the hills immediately above, from whence can be seen as usual an extensive and beautiful view.

Our last visit to these gardens was late in the autumn, one evening at sunsetting; their aspect changed, but the golden tints on tree and bower contrasting with the deep crimson of the autumn roses rather increased than diminished their beauty. One night too we visited them by moonlight, and the scene was one of unearthly beauty. Bebek was so easy of access from Koulali that we often went across, and the muses used to be very fond of visiting these gardens, and we were glad to find occasional amusement for them.

It is said there is an old Turkish superstition that no man dies while he is building a house, and that this is one reason why the *Sultans* of Turkey have built such innumerable palaces; no one content with those raised by his ancestors, but each new sovereign commencing some new work. Up to this time, however, all the royal buildings have been made of wood, believing that it was good enough for man, while stone was only fit for the temples of God.

But Abdul Medid has broken through the custom, and is building for himself a magnificent palace of marble immediately above Constantinople. It is called *Dolmabaghdshah*, or the filled-up garden. It forms one of the finest objects in the scenery of the Bosphorus; its extent is very great. Along the whole front runs a marble terrace, bordered with pillars and grating of finely-wrought iron, richly gilded.

The principal gateway is in the centre of this terrace, and there are several side entrances from all of which lead flights of marble steps, whose foundation rests in the water.

There used to be even more difficulty in the Franks gaining admission to view this palace than in other Turkish buildings, but those times are passed, and the allies have broken down the barrier—nothing more is needed than to go under the escort of an officer whose uniform and sword, accompanied of course with *backshish*, throw open the doors.

We disembarked at one side entrance; the grand entrance being reserved expressly for the *Sultan*. We entered the grand hall in which the *Sultan* holds his audience. The *coup d'oeil* was grand—rich gilding, *fresco* painting, and marble pillars presented a splendid scene. But the first effect was almost all; and with a nearer view the illusion vanishes, and the true Turkish architecture is clearly to be discerned, for general effect, with total absence of good detail, is its characteristic. The marble pillars were but painted wood! while a close view into every detail gave such an impression of rudeness and imperfection that we soon gave up the examination.

We ascended to the upper apartments, and were struck by another hall surmounted with a dome of ruby glass. The effect of this we liked exceedingly; the white marble of this hall was neither gilded nor painted, but only lit up with this deep glow. The effect was dazzling, reminding one rather of the hall in Aladdin's palace than any building belonging to this "work-a-day world." Almost all the innumerable apartments of the *Sultan*, for there are hundreds of them, are ornamented with fresco paintings.

The principal devices are of flowers, which gives a great sameness; the reason of this is that the *Koran* forbids the representation of any human or animal life, bestowing on those who disobey the curse of hereafter giving an account of the souls of those whose bodies they had thus dared to represent on earth. Another disappointment was, with the exception of the two halls, the extreme smallness of the regal apartments. Instead of constructing extensive ones, the space is broken up in continuous small rooms opening into each other.

The Imperial Haréem is separated from the other part of the palace by a corridor and garden. Upon entering we were instantly struck with the extreme contrast to the splendour of the other part of the palace. With a few exceptions, the rooms were perfectly plain, and the bed-rooms resembled those of a modern London house.

The *sultana's* drawing-room was, however, very prettily ornamented, and hung with innumerable glass chandeliers. We observed the introduction of a number of chairs in addition to the universal divan. One room, apparently set apart for study, was papered with deep crimson, the curtains and furniture of the same colour, chairs richly gilt; bureau and escritoire of polished wood were placed in different parts of the room; a pair of small globes stood on the table—all this evidently of Parisian workmanship.

But the gem of the palace is yet to be described—this was the *Sultan's* bath. We passed through a series of marble cooling rooms till we reached the bath. It is entirely of pale yellow alabaster, a kind rarely seen and difficult to procure. The roof was, of course, pierced to allow the vapour to escape; the sculpture is magnificent, and executed with the most delicate precision. There are several fountains, which, when the bath is heated, will pour forth rose-water.

The palace is not yet completed, though many of the rooms are completely furnished. The *Sultan* comes here daily at two p.m. to receive his officers of state; after this hour, therefore, no visitors are admitted. The Turk who conducted us over the palace seemed anxious to impress upon our minds the awful consequence of incurring the displeasure of the *Sultan* by speaking too loud or making the slightest sound. Upon our entrance he declared we must take off our shoes; we did not feel inclined to walk over all the marble floors without them, and resisted; and, after some discussion, additional *backshish* prevailed on him to waive the point as regarded the ladies, and he only insisted that the gentlemen of the party should slip huge Turkish slippers over their boots.

He walked first on tip-toe, putting his finger to his mouth, and when we talked or laughed, he drew his arm across his throat, saying, "*Sooltan, Sooltan,*" intimating that we had better take care of our heads. He seemed much entertained, though somewhat aghast at our extreme indifference to this warning. He evidently thought our continued laughing and talking a proof of wonderful courage; in fact, it so much excited his admiration, that on parting from him at the door of the palace, he made us understand that he would have no objection to *cicerone* us on a future occasion.

The garden was too formal and shrubless to attract our attention; it is laid out in numerous flower beds. The view from the windows is, as usual from buildings on the Bosphorus, exceedingly magnificent.

Chapter 21

The Crescent and the Cross

Papafée, out strange interpreter, who has been already mentioned, did not improve as time went on. We were often on the point of dismissing him and seeking another servant, but he used to go to Lady Stratford and talk her over, and, much to our astonishment, she expressed her wish that he should remain. He was a real annoyance, and, had it not been for the sake of his wife, who was a great comfort in sickness, we must have insisted on his removal. He used to scold us, tell falsehoods, offer his advice when quite unasked and unwished for; sometimes refused to do what he was told, and, when he did condescend to be obedient, let us fully understand that he was good enough to bend his superior judgment to our want of sense.

If we seriously offended him, he would threaten to write to England and report us to government. His whole conduct was so utterly absurd that we had many a laugh about it, and had these scenes only occurred now and then they would have been rather an amusement than otherwise, but with our various occupations and many calls, both on time and patience, this could not always be the case.

Papafée's wife was a little German woman, extremely gentle and quiet, and was the very opposite of her husband, who used to scold her loudly and severely if she the least displeased him, which was not a difficult matter to accomplish, and one of daily occurrence, though it was generally quite unintentional on her part; added to which she was much out of health, and needed kindness and attention. One of our ladies remonstrated with him on the subject.

"It ees very easy for you to talk," replied he; "you are an English lady, and it comes natural to you to be verie gentle and quiet, and you do say 'pleese do thees, and pleese do that,' but as for me I am of a deeferent deesposition. I was born in a deeferent contree, and am verie passionate, and beesides I can reed the Bible, and I do see there that the wife is to obey her husband, and that he ees to rule over her."

"Yes," replied the lady, "but the Bible also says husbands are to be kind to their wives."

"Oh, vell," said he, "so I am—I am verie kind indeed to her. You should jist see what beauteeful dresses I do give her. I do assure you they are verie fine. In my own contree I am quite a gentleman, and I could have married any lady I chose. My wife was verie luckee to get mee for her husband." This was an opinion in which no one shared, however, not even poor Rosalie herself.

Happily, for us we heard one day that our interpreter was wanted by a gentleman proceeding to the camp, who would give him better pay than he received from us. We were only too glad to release him, and he accordingly went up to the front, leaving his wife and child with us till he could make arrangements for them to join him.

Two months passed away, when one evening as we were all sitting at tea in our dining-room, which, opened to the garden, we saw coming down the path a tall, distinguished-looking officer. We wondered who it could be. To our surprise, instead of calling the servant he walked straight into the room, *sans cérémonie*. I thought he was some official come on important business from General Storks. Walking up to the head of the table, and making a low bow to our superintendent, he "hoped we were all well, and was glad to see us again," and not till then did we recognise our former plague and interpreter, Monsieur Papafée.

He then informed us that he was doing very well in the camp, and had come to fetch his wife and child, thinking Madame Papafée would turn a penny up there cooking for the officers. His appearance altogether was really so striking and elegant that we asked one another was it possible he had ever stood behind our chairs in white shirt sleeves and apron, or that we had ever asked him for a plate?

The next day one of us, returning from the hospital, saw a lady and gentleman walking arm-in-arm on the quay, followed by a servant carrying a child. On approaching them it proved to be Monsieur and Madame Papafée, whom we imagined he had ordered to deck herself for the occasion in one of the beautiful dresses he had once alluded to, as proving his devoted affection to the poor little woman. He made a polite bow as the lady passed.

They went to the camp, but not long afterwards, when walking in Pera, one of us was suddenly accosted by Papafée, who said he had left his situation at Sebastopol because, although it was very nice to be well paid, it was anything but agreeable to have a cannon ball coming into one's tent at all hours of the day or night; and a shell having burst in close proximity to his abode he had forthwith packed up and departed, agreeing no doubt with the old proverb, which says that in this world "*good people are scarce.*"

He was anxious to return to the "Home," but, fortunately, we did not need his services, for after his departure to the camp a friend had kindly recommended us a young Greek lad as servant. His name was Georgie. He was a great improvement upon Papafée, though not quite so talented as that remarkable individual. This, however, was amply compensated for, by his obedience and extreme anxiety to give us satisfaction. A Greek boy's dress is striking; the full loose trousers, gathered in at the knee, the striped pink cotton shirt, Tartar scarf round the waist, deep blue jacket, crimson *fez*, white stockings and polished shoes, is altogether very picturesque.

Georgie's language was a mixture of Greek, Turkish, Italian, French, and a few words of English. His eagerness to understand what we said was most amusing. If we asked for anything he stood looking at us very earnestly—his black eyes wide open and his finger in his mouth as if they would help him to understand our meaning. Sometimes he would shake his head and say, "No understands, missie; Georgie no speak much English!" But if happy enough to catch the meaning, his eyes would sparkle and he would dart off like an arrow to execute his commission.

One of our party was anxious to copy some hymn tunes used in the little hospital church. We had no piano, but the wife of one of the civilian doctors kindly offered us the use of hers whenever we had time to walk to her house at Candalee. To accomplish this, we had to climb some very steep hills, and as it was not safe to go alone the lady told Georgie to get ready to accompany her.

"Ah, *bono mademoiselle*," said Georgie, "very good, indeed!" with a look of intense delight, and off he ran.

In half an hour he returned, dressed in full holiday attire.

"Ah, Georgie, how smart you look!"

"Ah, *mademoiselle*, Georgie go with you; very good, much pleasure, so Georgie make himself smart."

She set out, followed by her very amusing page, who united the respectful manners of an English servant with the simplicity and affection of a child.

The road to Candalee is for some distance along a narrow path, on each side of which are houses in a continuous line; it then winds up the hill, which is extremely steep, and without shade; the full glare of the sun, therefore, falls upon one.

At last, they reached the summit of the hill and descended into a ravine. Georgie's delight seemed to increase till, as we passed a vineyard full of beautiful grapes, in he rushed and began vigorously gathering the best bunches, asking the lady to take as many as she pleased.

"No, no, Georgie," replied she; "come away quick—you very naughty—grapes not yours."

"Yes, yes, *signora*," cried he, "me quite good; they my bruder's grapes; he live other side hill up there; you come see him by and bye; he like you take plenty no pay, all *complimento*." He gathered bunch after bunch.

She thought it very odd, but having become accustomed to odd things in Turkey ceased to remonstrate, only begging him to make haste. He led her through the vineyard and up the next hill where, sure enough, was a little cottage, or rather shed, where he said his "bruder" lived, who it appears kept a vineyard and sold grapes at Constantinople or in the neighbourhood. Georgie made her sit down, and then fetched his bruder and seester—she appearing to be about sixty, and he, seventy years of age. Georgie was about eighteen.

"These are your father and mother, are they not?" said the lady.

"Oh no, my *pater* is *morto*," said Georgie, pointing to the ground.

"These my bruder and seester, *signora*."

We suppose they were in reality his aunt and uncle; they were most polite and kind, offering figs, melons, and grapes, and urging their visitor to partake of some, and take the rest home with her.

The whole scene was most picturesque—the young Greek boy in his holiday dress, and the old man and woman with their Eastern hospitality. After resting awhile, with many thanks the lady went her way, and, after copying the music, returned home—Georgie having employed the time during which he was waiting for her in making bouquets for her and the other ladies at the Home. One great pleasure of these Greek boys was to present us with flowers; they were very grateful and affectionate, and so pleased with any little present we gave them, which they always called "*complimento.*"

One day Miss—— gave Georgie a small print of the Crucifixion; he walked about the garden kissing it and pressing it to his heart. On another occasion he was ill in bed with a very bad foot; he slept in a small shed adjoining the Home. Miss —— took him some copies of the *Illustrated News* to amuse him, only intending to lend them, Georgie then expressed his thanks by kissing her hand, evidently taking it for a "*complimento;*" and behold the next day the walls of his room were adorned with the sheets of the *Illustrated News* pasted all over them!

Ramazan commenced in June; it lasts thirty days. The Turks fast till sunset, both from eating, drinking, and smoking; the two latter privations make it very hard work, as ordinarily a Turk never has his pipe from his lips, and the heat causes great thirst. Shortly before sunset the Turkish troops assemble in the barrack-yard with their large copper dishes; rice is portioned out to them, sometimes mixed with a sort of gravy, and they stand still looking at it till the welcome sound of the sunset gun (which is fired the moment the sun sinks below the horizon) is heard, and then they set to with good appetites to enjoy their dirty-looking dinner.

The *caidjees* greatly object to taking passengers when near sunset time, but if persuaded to do so and the gun is heard they will stop at the nearest village to get their pipes lighted before they will proceed.

After sunset throughout *Ramazan* all peace and quiet is over. After the Turks have done eating, they begin shouting and dancing and what they call music, a sound resembling that which would be produced in England by one hundred hurdy-gurdies, all playing together. The noise is distracting, and generally lasts until two or three in the morning. It was annoying even to those in the Home, but the officers, whose quarters were close beside the Turkish barracks, complained bitterly of the impossibility of sleeping in consequence of it. All were thankful when the fast drew to its close.

Some of the English residents advised us strongly not to lose the sight of Bairam or Beiram, the Great Feast which follows *Ramazan*. This was a matter of difficulty, living the distance we did from Constantinople, but through the kindness of friends some of our party were able to have the enjoyment.

The ceremonies of Beiram are as follows: The *Sultan* must be in Santa Sophia at sunrise, after which he receives in the gardens of his *seraglio* his Ministers of State and the chief men of the empire. There are two feasts called by this name commanded to be observed by Mahomet—the first, or the Greater Bairam, is kept at Mecca only when victims are sacrificed, and it is called by the Arabs "*Id al Korbam, il al adha*," *i.e.*, "The Feast of the Sacrifice," which is celebrated in memory of the sacrifice of Abraham.

But the feast we were about to witness is called the Lesser Bairam, or in Arabia, "*Id al Feti*." It is dependent on the new moon; if the sky is so cloudy that she cannot be discerned, the feast is postponed for one day, but after that it proceeds whether they see her or not. Watchers are placed on the surrounding hills to catch the first glimpse of her appearance, and then they run to the city, crying, "Welcome news," and the festivity commences.

We were obliged to quit Koulali at two a.m., to reach Stamboul in time. *Caiques* were engaged, and the Turkish sergeant-major volunteered to go as interpreter. This worthy was a remarkable character in the hospital. He prided himself on his knowledge of English, small though it certainly was. He took the opportunity of our row down the Bosphorus to inquire into the manners and customs of England—to ask about the pay of English sergeant-majors—to inform us that his own was sixpence a-day—to say that he admired the English more than the Turks, and intended to visit that country and enter its service, and indeed his anxiety to visit England was so great that he offered himself to us in the capacity of cook , if we would only take him.

The grimaces he made, and his gesticulations with his broken English, and his excessive amusement at our few Turkish words was like this, "English very *bono*; Turk no *bono*; English soldier how much? Turk soldier so much; I go you? hidi England; I you cook; ship hidi Angleterre; very *bono*," and so on.

The night was very dark, but as our *caiques* glided down the Bosphorus the banks were continually illuminated by the flashes of firearms which were incessantly fired from the batteries on the hills and from the *Sultan's* numerous palaces. So continual was this discharge that the Bosphorus was a blaze of light. As one flash died away another sprang up, and the hills gave back the echo of the cannon's thunder.

As we approached Stamboul the morning had begun to dawn. The first rays of the sun gilded the imperial city. We were not there yet. We had to pass through the Golden Horn and disembark near Seraglio Point. It was my first visit to Stamboul or Istamboul, as it is rightly called, and what a flood of memories of the "old historic page" came over me as I felt I was about to enter this ancient and far-famed city! How the long train of her eventful history rose before my mind!

First one's thoughts wandered back to old Byzantium and her mighty fortifications, when her walls were as though of one single block, 1263 years before Christ, so lost in the mist of ages we can hardly trace it; but we know well those old walls withstood many a shock. Siege and assault were matters full of interest to us, and we remembered the walls and the towers, and the showers of stones which greeted the besiegers, and, lastly, the cables of the ships woven of the women's hair. Alas! we doubt whether the patriotism of modern ladies would carry them thus far.

Years pass on and Byzantium becomes a Christian city. Constantine the Great sits on the imperial throne; the idol temples are thrown down; the old walls ring with Christian worship. The Cross by which Constantine conquered stands in the public places. Byzantium was a name that passed away, and the conqueror named the city after his own name Constantinople, and he forsakes even Rome for his new possession. Constantine averred it was by the especial command of Heaven that he traced out the walls of the new city. Nocturnal visions had guided him. On foot, lance in hand, and followed by a long procession, the emperor marked out the boundaries, and the astonished people at length observed that he had already exceeded the most ample measure of a great city.

"I shall still advance," said Constantine, "till He the invisible Guide who marches before me thinks proper to stop."

Years passed on. The long line of Constantines fill the throne. What scenes of strife and bloodshed went on within those old walls! Five hundred years after Constantine had died, the storm of the great schism is heard. Then the Ottoman power advances, attacks, makes visible inroads into the great empire, till at last, in 1453, the Mussulman reigns in that proud city.

And now our *caique* touches the quay, and we come back to the realities of Turkish life in 1855, not so much unlike 1453 as might he supposed. We left our *caiques* and walked about a mile to the open plain before the *Seraglio*, where the *Sultan* was staying, and from whence he would pass to Santa Sophia. Stamboul was all alive. *Pashas* with their trains were busily riding hither and thither. A large body of Turkish troops were drawn up in the square awaiting His Majesty. Visitors of all nations swelled the throng.

We waited here about an hour, amusing ourselves by walking up and down and watching the evolutions of the *pashas* on horseback. The enormous size of some of the *pashas* made the management of their steeds a matter of difficulty. They certainly gave one the impression of a considerable falling off from the courage of their great ancestors, whose valour was such that neither Cyrus nor Alexander could conquer them. Judging by the streets, manufactories, and public buildings of the city the genius of their great father Turk, the son of Japhet, from whom they so proudly trace their origin, has vanished too.

Now the procession began to form. First came three or four carriages, containing the *sultanas* and other ladies very gaily attired. Now the *Sultan's* horses were led out, their trappings of embroidered silk and jewels; then came many a *pasha* with his train. At length the "Commander of the Faithful," surrounded by his guards, and on horseback. He was dressed in uniform, over which was thrown a cloak of dark blue cloth, fastened by a buckle of brilliants; he wore the crimson *fez*, in which was a plume of heron's feathers, secured by a diamond clasp. The simplicity of his dress formed a striking contrast to his magnificently attired *pashas'*.

Slowly the procession passed to Santa Sophia—the Turkish troops cheering the *Sultan* as he proceeded along the line in deep solemn tones, very unlike the hearty, joyous cheering of our own land. A dense mass of people followed. We reached the entrance of the mosque, and beheld the floor entirely covered with Turks all prostrate with their foreheads on the ground. The *imauns* at the door furiously refused admittance to Franks. One naval officer had contrived to slip in, and, in answer to all their violent gesticulations, held up his shoes with an earnest look to let them see how *much* he had sacrificed to their prejudices, and he kept his place, for they dared not lay violent hands on an officer in uniform.

No wonder they did not want any Franks if they really followed the universal custom at Beiram, and prayed either for the rooting out of all Christian princes, or that they might quarrel among themselves. It would be curious if they prayed in 1855 for the overthrow of Queen Victoria, Louis Napoleon, and Victor Emanuel; perhaps they thought, provided Alexander went too, it did not much signify if the Allies accompanied him.

Owing to our being accompanied by an officer we gained admittance to the *seraglio* gardens, and saw the *Sultan* pass through them on his return to the palace. We waited there about an hour while he took some refreshment. A throne was now placed immediately before the palace covered with crimson velvet; a carpet of the same material at its foot. An open space was cleared, around which were ranged troops. Opposite the throne was the royal band, and we and other strangers ranged ourselves behind the soldiers.

It was a beautiful "presence chamber"—those lovely gardens, and beneath the shade of the old green trees—the cloudless summer sky for his canopy, to receive his Court in. Several ladies and numbers of French and English officers stood around. Conspicuous amongst them was Monsieur Soyer, whose costume always marked him out.

At last, the *Sultan* appeared; he walked up ungracefully to his throne and seated himself. We were in a position to get an excellent view of him and of the whole proceedings. He is a thin, pale, dark, wearied-looking man, giving one the impression of a person void of energy, and who would fain be rid of a heavy burden.

As soon as he was seated, the *pashas* began to walk before him in procession—some kissing their sovereign's hand, others only bowing low to the ground before him; then the *beys* followed in order. The *pashas* and *beys* were all in European dress, with the exception of the crimson *fez*; but their dresses were covered with rich embroidery. Then came the *imauns*, hundreds of them, of different degrees and rank. All bowed low before him, making the *salaam, i.e.,* putting their right hand first to their forehead, then to their breast, and bending their heads nearly to the ground.

Some of these, apparently of higher rank or dignity, kissed the *Sultan's* feet, or rather the hem of his robe; others merely kissed the fringe of a long scarf which was passed over his shoulders, and held by one of his chief officers at some little distance from the royal person.

Whenever the *imauns*, dressed in the sacred green (the descendants of Mahomet) approached, the *Sultan* rose and extended his hand for them to kiss, which they did with the utmost reverence. He continued standing quite erect till they passed out of his sight. The whole scene was most striking, nearly all the *imauns* being dressed in different colours—white, red, yellow, or green, in all their shades—and the last in blue, the only one wearing that colour. All wore a high white turban, except the descendants of the Prophet, who were dressed entirely in green, turban and all.

During the pauses in the procession, which sometimes occurred, the Turkish band played; and, although the music was very inferior to that heard in our own land, yet it sounded rather sweetly that early morning in the beautiful *seraglio* gardens and added greatly to the romance of the whole scene. When they had all passed, which was not till about eight o'clock a.m., the *Sultan* rose and departed as ungracefully as he had entered, not even bowing to those around. The festivity of Beiram lasts three days, and incessant firing of cannon goes on day and night.

The assembly broke up, and we were not sorry; for the fatigue of six hours' standing, after a sleepless night, was very great. When we reached our *caiques*, the sun had become glaringly hot, and making our voyage home a most disagreeable one; so that we could hardly listen to the incessant conversation of the sergeant-major, who now quite changed his tone, and did nothing but extol the greatness of Turkey, its *Sultan*, and *pashas*.

CHAPTER 22

The Nuns' Careful Nursing

The heat at the end of July grew intense, and continued so till the end of the following month. Up to this time it had been like a very warm English summer; but now the Eastern sun poured down all its fury upon us, and we were terribly exposed to its rays. No kind of shade was at hand: there was hardly a tree in Koulali. The five minutes' walk from our home to hospital, was along the quay.

The Sisters of Mercy, who came down from the General Hospital and returned thither twice a-day, had to descend and climb the steep hill in the glaring sun; so, also, the ladies who worked at the General Hospital. Our hospital duties obliged us to be walking about during the greater part of the time when the inhabitants of the country close their *jalousies* and take their *siesta*, not venturing to move till sunset.

The heat was real suffering; it brought incessant thirst, which nothing could quench. The quantity of lemonade which was drank during that time was something marvellous, and it seemed impossible to touch the meat of the country; and yet too great a quantity of acid, and the omission of strengthening food, was considered very dangerous, as likely to bring on cholera.

We feared that cholera would have been very prevalent in the summer—thank God it was not so!—twenty was the utmost of those attacked, and out of these not more than half were fatal. At the General Hospital were several bad cases, whose lives were saved, humanly speaking, by the attention they received from the nuns, who watched by them day and night.

A great blessing arrived about this period, in the shape of ice; it was sent out by government. The ship that brought it was called the *City of Montreal*, her captain was a Scotchman; he purchased a cargo of ice in North America at a venture, which proved a fortunate one, for three days after coming into Liverpool the whole was bought by government, and he was instantly despatched with it to the East. Part was left at Scutari, part at Koulali, the rest went to Balaclava. The captain reckoned he had made £500 by the enterprise. Thankful indeed were we that he had made it.

There was an ice-house at the General Hospital into which the ice was put, and we used to send the Greeks to fetch it down to the Barrack. Unfortunately, the ice-house was not a good one, and the ice melted faster than it would otherwise have done; so, we were obliged to use it as fast as possible, but it lasted the exact time the extreme heat did. I cannot think what we should have done without it. Certainly, we could not have given "cooling drinks" any longer, for the lemonade used to be quite warm till iced; and it was such a comfort to the fever patients to lay on their burning brows, and most useful in cholera; also, in obstinate cases of diarrhoea and dysentery it checked vomiting and allayed the irritation of the stomach.

There were two cases of cholera in the Barrack Hospital which were remarkable; they were in different wards, one in the surgical the other in the dysentery; their symptoms were exactly similar, consisting chiefly in extreme depression; they resisted all nourishment and wept almost incessantly, and no one could discover that they had any particular cause for grief. Both these cases were fatal.

Smoking was ordered in the wards when cholera was about; this was rather amusing to the men as they had been before strictly forbidden to smoke in the wards, and it had been a great deprivation to those not able to walk into the barrack-yard, for unless a man were in a dying state, he had strength enough for his beloved pipe; even while it was forbidden, they would smoke whenever they could do so without being seen.

Another misery brought by the heat was the increase of vermin. Mosquitos began to pay us a visit; they never abounded so much as we expected, but they were quite bad enough, and their bite was very painful and disfiguring. We had mosquito-net from the stores, which we cut into squares and threw it over the faces of those who were very ill.

Fleas abounded and were very tormenting; we used a powder which can be bought at Stampa's shop in Galata, and to all Eastern travellers I should recommend it; for though it does not destroy these enemies, it stupefies them, and one has the satisfaction of seeing the sheets spread with them fast asleep, while otherwise the wretches are so very rapid in their movements that it is almost a hopeless undertaking to wage war against them. From their facility in making their escape, someone named them the "light cavalry," while *other horrors* which we occasionally had the misfortune to encounter in the wards, who were not so light of foot, were called "heavy dragoons."

The ice ship lay off Koulali for several days. The captain used to send his boat in the evening to know if we would like to have a row, and as it held a great many, we were glad to take the nurses out in it. When the *City of Montreal* was ready to proceed to Balaclava it was proposed that two or three ladies should go on board of her as far as the entrance to the Black Sea, and return in the steamer which would tug her up to that point. She was to start at six a.m.

We went on board one lovely morning; the steamer began to tug the vessel, but could not succeed. The current was so strong that she was powerless, and after trying for two hours in vain she was obliged to give it up. The steamers used for tugging are the small ones which ply upon the Bosphorus and are hired by the Admiralty. The *City of Montreal* was tugged up next day by the *Ottawar*, a fine steamship.

We did not attempt to see the Black Sea a second time, having been so disappointed the first day, so we contented ourselves with having seen the Euxine from Therapia without actually passing into its waters.

One day a ship came alongside Koulali wharf to coal; she had on board a Dr. Thompson and his wife. Dr. Thompson was a civilian, who had practised for some years in Antioch, before that I think in India, and was well known for scientific discoveries.

It appeared that he had wished to visit Balaclava, and had proceeded thither, accompanied by his wife; while there—living on board ship—was seized with the Crimean fever. When the ship was obliged to return, he was too ill to be moved, and indeed at Balaclava there was no place for him. The vessel came to Scutari, and application was made to the authorities for his admission into the hospital.

An unfortunate delay arose about granting this, which no doubt would have been done at length. The vessel could not wait; having discharged her cargo for Scutari she came to Koulali, Dr. Thompson still on board. The same application was made at Koulali, and was instantly granted; Koulali being a much smaller place than Scutari it had probably not to go through so many hands before it was decided on. At all events they were received.

The heat was so intense that though it was granted at noon they were forced to wait till the cool evening before they dared move him—for he was raving in delirium, and his fever was in the highest stage. Meanwhile, an empty ward in the General Hospital was prepared for his use, and everything which the hospital possessed in the way of comfort placed at his disposal by Dr. Humphrey, P. M. O. Our Superintendent appointed one of her best nurses to aid Mrs. Thompson in attending on him, and committed him also to the care of the Reverend Mother.

From that day for weeks the one topic of the hospital was Dr. Thompson. If he had been a king more could not have been done for him; his delirium was very violent, and he would take dislikes to the surgeons and want new ones. Accordingly, almost everyone in the hospital went to him at any time he chose to ask for them. He appeared to be fond of music, and it was thought singing would soothe him. One of the ladies accordingly went and sang to him for hours.

The Sisters of Mercy were most unremitting in their attentions, especially the Reverend Mother, who was called up night after night, and who cheerfully hastened to see if she could in any way relieve him. Fatigue and distress had their effect upon poor Mrs. Thompson, her grief was violent, and she required much attention. The Reverend Mother spent much time in soothing her, sometimes reading a few verses of the Holy Scriptures or a hymn. Mrs. Thompson spoke of her kindness afterwards with much gratitude.

Dr. Thompson and his wife were members of the Church of England. The chaplain visited them constantly, and he also used to be called up in the night when the delirium was at its height that he might endeavour to quiet the sufferer.

There was at one time a slight hope of his recovery, but an abscess, which was a frequent result of the Crimean fever, gathered in his neck, and death fast approached. The nurse who had been waiting on him, being worn out, returned to rest. Another whom we thought well of took her place, and a few hours after worse symptoms appeared.

Word of this being brought to the lady superintendent, she went at 11 p.m. to the General Hospital to see him. Upon entering the room, the scene was awful. He was in his last agony, his wife was by his side doing all she believed best for him. On a bed that had been standing in the room lay the nurse in a state of dead intoxication. She had, while passing from the Home to the hospital (the emergency having obliged her to be sent alone), purchased the Turkish spirits, which produce a perfect stupor. She could not be awakened, and the superintendent was obliged to call four orderlies to carry her upstairs, where she lay for hours in the same state.

All through the night the superintendent watched beside the sick bed. The chaplain came and read the commendatory prayers, and finding reason was not likely to return then left him. At Mrs. Thompson's desire the Presbyterian chaplain afterwards came and prayed beside him, and about 3 p.m. he expired.

His body was interred the following day in Koulali British burying-ground; all the medical staff followed in uniform.

Many of the ladies and nurses also attended to accompany his widow, whose wish it was to be present.

During life Dr. Thompson had often expressed a wish to be buried beneath a tree, and in sight of a beautiful view. There was but one tree in the burying-ground; under that they dug his grave, while all around lay spread one of the most beautiful scenes one could imagine.

During the whole summer only one case of serious illness occurred amongst our party. Miss F—— lay for many weeks ill with dysentery. She was attended by Dr. Guy, and to his extreme attention and skill, under God's blessing, she owed her recovery. After a time, she resumed her work. There was a great deal of sickness amongst us, though not of a serious character, but almost all suffered from the heat extremely.

In our illnesses we were attended only by the army surgeons, and they were kind beyond measure. About this time, to our great regret, Dr. Temple joined the Turkish Contingent; there was great mourning among his patients at his departure, for he was one of the kindest as well as the most skilful of the surgeons.

Chapter 23
Frequent Fires in Constantinople

One day we received a letter from Miss Stanley, with an account of an interview she had had with the queen, who sent for her and inquired with the deepest interest into the details of our work, and wished to know what more she could send out to contribute to the comfort of the sick and to assure them of her continual sympathy. The interview lasted near an hour, and at its close Her Majesty expressed her satisfaction at what she had heard, and her thanks for the service rendered. Miss Stanley also received the thanks of Prince Albert and the Duchess of Kent on a subsequent occasion.

She transmitted the royal thanks to us, feeling, as she said, she had only received them as the representative of all who had done the work.

In the royal gifts which came out a short time afterwards, we recognised the articles which Miss Stanley had named in answer to Her Majesty's inquiries. The pleasure these gifts of Her Majesty gave was immense; they consisted of a large quantity of raspberry jam, treacle, tamarinds, and pickles. Also, chess, dominoes, and draughts.

The gifts were valuable in themselves, but how much more so the remembrance of the thoughtful sympathy that had sent them out.

"Only to think of our queen thinking of such things for the like of us," said the patients.

But they had already grown familiar with the knowledge that the sufferings of the soldiers in camp and hospital were no less remembered in the palace than in their humble homes.

In all the wards was posted upon the walls the beautiful letter written by Queen Victoria to Mr. Sidney Herbert in the month of December 1854, and which caused such a thrill of gratitude and delight among the soldiers.

The *Illustrated London News*, which were distributed among them, had shown them how their queen "visited the sick." They saw her passing through hospital wards and speaking gentle words to the sufferers there. They heard of her warm interest in all they did or suffered, and that no hand but her own was allowed to decorate their comrades who had returned home.

The royal gifts were divided by the purveyor-in-chief, among the different Eastern hospitals. Pickles were only allowed by the medical officers for the convalescent patients, for whom doubtless Her Majesty intended them. Jam and treacle were used in all the wards; the latter many men preferred to butter; but the portion of the royal gifts which gave most delight were the chess, dominoes, and draughts.

The authorities of course informed Her Majesty of the gratitude and delight with which her bounty had been received; but those official letters told her but a small part. We often wished the queen could have once seen what we saw daily; the groups of men gathered round the table at those games, the extreme pleasure they gave them, the time they innocently employed, and the temptations of drink and idle company from which they kept them.

For ourselves, these royal gifts were not without a peculiar pleasure, as it showed us plainly that Her Majesty did not esteem common necessaries enough for her gallant army, but was determined that comforts, and even a few luxuries, should be poured upon them, and that she approved of our efforts to bring these to the men. Cheering to us in that far off land and amidst our many difficulties was the kind sympathy of our beloved queen.

Every traveller to Constantinople has spoken of the frequent fires. I do not know whether they were more numerous than usual this summer; but certainly, they were almost incessant. People said that at times it was done on purpose, the *Sultan* wishing to destroy some of the dirty wooden houses; but I think this is improbable. They generally occurred at night. We always knew they were going on by the firing of seven guns from the Turkish battery on the hill above Koulali. Sometimes we rose and looked, for the sight was very fine; but at last, they grew so frequent that they hardly roused us.

One night a discharge of cannon was heard. I had grown so used to it, that I concluded it was the first of the seven guns, and did not disturb myself. A noise in the house attracted my attention. I rose, and, going into the corridor, found the whole household assembled and gazing out of the corridor windows with looks of alarm. Apparently, the General Hospital was on fire. Our first thought was for the Sisters of Mercy: the patients, we knew, would be carried to the Barrack Hospital; but the Sisters would be homeless.

Two of us dressed in haste, and went out. As we approached the foot of the hill, a body of troops rushed down. They perceived us, and a sergeant stopped to inform us that some gunpowder, kept in a shed not far from the General Hospital, had taken fire and exploded, which was the sound we heard.

No danger had occurred, and no lives were lost, though, on the first alarm, all the troops, British and Turkish, were turned out; and the sergeant declared he was asleep, dreaming Sebastopol was taken, and when the sudden call came, he thought it was to summon him to the assault.

We hastened home to quell the anxiety of our companions; and the alarm over, the laughing began, as we who had been out declared they all looked like Turkish ladies in *feridgees*, sitting on the divan of the corridor.

When the day came, we went to congratulate the Sisters on their escape. They said they had been much alarmed, the explosion being so very near their apartments; and when they were awakened by the sudden noise, and immediately afterwards the tramp of the troops coming up the hill, one of them confessed she thought the Russians had come! at which we all laughed very much.

One morning when we came down to prayers, we saw a fire on the opposite coast. The villages are so thickly joined together that we could hardly distinguish where it was. It was a palace of the *Sultan*, said to belong to the *Sultan's* Sister. If it was this palace, one was not sorry to see it burnt down; for horrible traditions attach to the name of Asma, Sultan Mahmoud's Sister; and, it is said, from underneath a low arch, bodies were often seen to float into the Bosphorus from her palace.

Whether it was her palace or not, it was in flames, and in half-an-hour was destroyed, for it was of course built of wood, and a strong breeze blew from the Black Sea, and the work of devastation was rapid.

Many houses stood near whose owners were in great alarm. Next to them came a grove of cypresses, and a large villa beyond them stood higher up the hill. Curiously enough the flames did not touch the adjoining houses. We thought when we saw the palace falling into pieces that its fury was spent, when suddenly behind the cypresses the forked flames burst out, catching the villa and destroying it. It is thus that the fires in Turkey spread, so that when they once begin the whole village often falls. In this case, however, when the villa was burnt the fire was arrested.

It was a striking sight to see the volume of bright flame behind those dark trees, which it did not attempt to touch, and lower down the hill the burning blackened ruins of the palace, falling piece by piece into the blue Bosphorus, while the lurid glare of the fire mingled with the bright sunshine of that cloudless summer morning.

During the summer the hospital library was established. A large room fitted with shelves was given for this purpose. It was under the charge of Mr. Coney, the Church of England chaplain. He requested the ladies would assist him in getting it into order.

The superintendent had no one whom she could send, so she added the charge to her own numerous duties. The task of sorting and arranging was a long and tedious one. Numbers of cases arrived and contained many nice books; but a quantity of rubbish among them, reports of charities, old encyclopaedias, &c., &c. Then would come most provoking *portions* of books; fragments of all the Waverley novels, with not one complete; odd numbers of ancient magazines.

Next would come a number of little books for Sunday scholars, which we certainly deemed as much below the capacity of the men as the number of essays on abstruse subjects which were sent were above them. A great many nice books came too. Mr. Albert Smith's handsome present had arrived long months before; but of course, many of his books furnished the library shelves.

The arrangement of the library was a great comfort. Before it was opened the books were kept in the chaplain's quarters; we used to go there and hunt through the cases for the kind we wanted. Now they were all arranged in order. Bibles and prayer-books by themselves, religious books in another part, instructive works in a third, and the novels and tales in a fourth; magazines by themselves, while those who wished to read the mutilated Waverley, &c. could find them on a top shelf.

There was a good store of Bibles and prayer-books, but we were always asking for more from England, as the chaplains gave them to each man not possessing them when he left either for home or camp.

The Catholic religious books were generally sent to the Catholic chaplain or Sisters. If they came into the library, they were forwarded to them. Five hundred Catholic Testaments were sent by kind friends, and were much valued. Other packets of books arrived, but many others shared the frequent fate of parcels to the East, and never reached their destination.

Several hundreds of Scotch Bibles with the Psalms, as used in the Kirk, came to the general library, and were forwarded by Mr. Coney to the Presbyterian chaplain for the exclusive use of his congregation.

Secular books were of course for all classes alike, and, after they had been sorted, the ladies and Sisters had free access to the library, and could take as many as they pleased. How the men did delight in those books! Every ward had a little lending library of its own, books taken from the general library, and lent and changed from one to another all round the ward. Books were sent out by the Duchess of Kent; amongst them were many copies of St. John's history of the present war which was a great favourite.

Chapter 24

The Religious Spirit in the British Army

There were three chaplains appointed to Koulali—the Church of England, the Catholic, and the Presbyterian (sometimes there were two of the first-mentioned). When the wards were so crowded no place was set apart for public worship, and the men being chiefly in their beds or unable to walk, it was only the men on duty who attended the services. At that time the English and Scotch services were held at respective hours on Sundays only, in the detachment ward in the morning or the convalescent hospital in the afternoon.

The Catholic services were daily in the Sisters' oratory in the General Hospital, where the men could attend, and on Sundays in the chaplain's own room in the Barrack Hospital; when the summer came on and it became evident that the new wards which had been fitted up in the winter would never all be filled, one was given to the English chaplain, a room in the General Hospital to the Catholic, and another empty ward in the Barrack to the Presbyterian.

The ward used for the English service was the one fronting the *Sultan's* apartments. The roof was sloping and not very high; it was very wide and would have made a fine ward. It was four times too large for its purpose, as the congregation only filled half one side.

Up to the time of Mr. Coney's arrival the services were only on Sundays (except Ash Wednesday and Good Friday). Soon after he became senior chaplain, he established daily morning prayers; and the communion, which had been administered monthly, was now given every Sunday at 7.30 a.m.

The purveyor-in-chief had the ward furnished with church fittings, and some of the ladies aided to beautify it, and it looked very nice when finished, though of course rudely adorned. The altar rails were of plain deal, a red cloth covered the table, and the reading-desk was hung with the same colour. A few benches were arranged on each side, some with backs to them were also placed lower down for the invalids, and the wooden trestles of the empty beds formed seats for the rest of the congregation.

This congregation on Sunday made a singular scene. The different groups: a number of men on duty in their uniforms, then a mass of fine dressing-gowns and white nightcaps, another of nurses in grey dresses, the ladies seated among them either in black or colours; on the other side the officers also in uniform, one or two officers' wives, and sometimes a few English strangers from the neighbouring village of Bebek, on the European side, the only Protestant service there being in the Protestant Armenian chapel, and the singing was so atrocious, they said, they preferred coming across to Koulali, where the singing was very good considering its difficulties.

There being no instrument it was led by one of the ladies who had a singing-class twice a-week, which the convalescent patients and some of the sergeants and detachment men attended. They were very fond of coming to it, and took great pains to learn the chants and hymn tunes; those they had been accustomed to hear in the churches at home pleased them most.

The Presbyterian service was at the same hour as the English one. The members of this congregation were fewer than either the English or Catholic churches. Two of the ladies of our party and one of the nurses belonged to it. Many of the Presbyterian soldiers appeared to be earnest and religious men. The chaplain was exceedingly active in visiting the sick members of his congregation.

The Catholic chapel was arranged with great taste, though of course with the greatest simplicity; the altar was raised on the divan, which fronted the windows. The room was furnished with benches, the middle space left for the men and officers, the Sisters kneeling on each side. A few coloured prints hung on the wall; every tiling was very rough, but all the essentials of Catholic worship were there. The services were well attended by the men. The two masses on Sundays (one at each hospital) were crowded; the daily mass had a good gathering, and so had the Sunday benediction.

The chaplain for many months was Mr. Ronan; this priest was most zealous and devoted, beloved by his flock, and respected by all. The improvement among the Catholics in Koulali was very great. The soldiers had been much neglected, and many had yielded to temptation, contracted evil habits, and forgotten their religion, but the efforts made by the priests and nuns were blessed. Those who had lived long years in sin once more sought their Saviour—those whose last remembrance of prayers and sacraments had been in days gone by, in the shelter of their homes, now returned to the God of their youth.

Were these pages the fitting place many a tale might be told of such, but they are not. It will, however, interest Catholics to hear that the Sisters of Mercy had the satisfaction of knowing that no member of their church ever left the hospitals of Koulali without receiving the sacraments, nor did any die without their consolations.

It will interest others to know among the members of the Church of England a marked improvement took place many turning from evil or careless lives and becoming earnest and zealous in religion, thus rewarding their good chaplain's labours, who spared no pains in the performance of his duty. When Mr. Coney established the daily morning prayers he expected them to be attended by about a dozen at the utmost. To his surprise and pleasure, he found more than that come even the first morning, and in a week's time it had increased to thirty or more. The time for prayers was half-past seven in the morning.

Beautiful indeed were those early mornings, before the glaring sun attained its power; the golden light adorning the distant white walls and towers of Constantinople with a crown of glory. It looked like a visionary city, making one think of the one for which "we seek," and which "is to come." The dewdrops sparkled on the grass, the clear sweet singing of the birds came through the open windows. The blue ripples of the Bosphorus shone brightly, and our first waking sensations were those of admiration of all this wonderful beauty. When we went out the air was so light and fresh and invigorating.

A little before seven in the morning a group of convalescents, dressed in blue, and soldiers in uniform, were seen climbing the hill to attend mass. Many who were very weak persisted in going, and counted the fatigue nothing in comparison of the blessing they would receive. At half-past seven another group wended their way to the English prayers.

When the heat was gone, and the work had very much diminished, the daily service was altered to nine in the morning, and when Dr. Freeth succeeded Mr. Coney as chaplain he established an evening one at six o'clock. These services were well attended both by officers and men, who chanted and sang very heartily at each of them. The officers seemed to prefer the later hour in the morning, as now the brunt of the work was over, they were not obliged to be in their wards so early as in the summer; this was also the case with some of the ladies and nurses.

These are plain proofs that the spirit of real religion is in the British army, and only needs culture to bring it out, and had not its spiritual wants been so grievously neglected it would not have become noted for its irreligion, nor would English parents have had cause hitherto to consider it a disgrace that their sons should fill its ranks. The following anecdotes will show how ready they were to amend. One orderly bore a very high character, and was much liked by the Sister of the award for his good conduct. One day he became intoxicated; when he came to his senses, he hid himself from the Sister. However, she met him accidentally and expressed her sorrow and displeasure; he had been a soldier for seventeen years, yet he blushed before her as a guilty schoolboy, and exclaimed—

"Oh, ma'am, look it over this time, it never shall happen again; I'd rather be summoned before all the doctors in the hospital and be punished by them, than that you should once reprove me."

Indeed, the orderlies at the Upper Hospital thought the Sisters' displeasure far worse than being sent to the guardroom.

One day an orderly, partly drunk when the Reverend Mother entered the ward, attempted to conceal his state; she turned away and called another, bidding the first go to bed at once. The next day he was ready as usual to carry round the extras for her. "No," she said, "you have disgraced yourself, I will have another." He slunk away ashamed. Some days passed, and she took no notice of him.

At last, one day he waylaid her in the corridor, where no one could hear him, and said with tears in his eyes, "Will you never forgive me, Reverend Mother? I am so miserable to be in disgrace with you—indeed I will amend for the future."

Chapter 25

Regimental and Camp Hospitals

Since June the numbers in the hospital had been gradually decreasing, and the character of the cases had completely changed. Of course, there were exceptions; but as a rule, those who came down from the front were nearly convalescent, needing only nourishment or change of air, and accordingly after they had been a few weeks in Koulali they were either invalided home or discharged to duty.

When the attack of the 18th of June took place, we looked for wounded and sick to come down, but not one arrived, and we then found that the medical and other authorities at head-quarters had determined to keep the sick as much as possible in the Crimea, considering the air there best for them, and the voyage down unadvisable.

The number of regimental hospitals had so increased that they were able to accommodate a large number. There was an hospital in the camp besides the General and Castle Hospitals, Balaclava, for the more serious cases. Besides, except from the attack of the 18th of June, the health of the army was far better than had been expected.

From these various causes arose the circumstance that the hospitals on the Bosphorus were more than half empty. Of course, this was a matter of great thankfulness, but the question arose whether our nursing staff was not too large for our work. As time went on, we became certain of this, and the accounts which the invalids and others brought from the Crimea, convinced us that the brunt of the work was passed from our hospitals and lay in the Crimea.

We knew that there were but few nurses there, and we were anxious that some of us should proceed there if required, a point we resolved to ascertain. Lord William Paulet was *commandant* at the time, and he had requested Lady Stratford de Redcliffe to exercise his authority over the nursing department. Our superintendent told Lady Stratford she was ready to go to the Crimea, but Lady Stratford negatived it at once, and in a decided manner. As no other lady was equal to the task of directing so untried and laborious an undertaking, the idea was relinquished.

The Reverend Mother soon after this writing to one of the chaplains, a friend of hers in the camp, told him how little we had to do in the hospital, and that she and the Sisters felt an earnest wish to have work such as they came to do. She read this letter to our superintendent, who agreed with its purport. The chaplain wrote in answer, that if she would again write and repeat her statements more formally, he would show it to Dr. Hall. The Reverend Mother did so, expressing in it how willing she would be either to continue under our present superintendent if it was thought desirable, or to go alone with her Sisters.

So, the matter rested, and we lived on in the usual state of uncertainty attending British affairs in the East. None but those who have experienced it could enter completely into this feeling. We hardly ever knew what had happened, or what was going to happen. Rumours of all kinds so continually buzzed about that, at last, we learned to believe nothing till we saw it in an English newspaper. The fall of Sebastopol we were told every week had taken place. Every imaginable tale was spread about.

The only incident just at this time was one which gave us some pleasure, in the departure of the Turkish troops stationed at the hospital. We were told the room was to be occupied with Sardinian soldiers. A quantity of boats came to fetch the Turks' baggage—there was a fine quantity of rubbish on the quay. The Turkish soldiers were a miserable-looking set, and we were glad to get rid of them; especially as we heard such a high character of the Sardinian soldiers.

Away the Turks went, but days went on and no Sardinians appeared. Then came in another tale. The Sardinians were badly off for room, especially for their sick. Three officers came one day, walked round our hospitals, and said, on seeing the convalescent hospital, "How happy we should be if we could only get this hospital for our poor sick."

Rumour now said that General Storks, who had by this time succeeded Lord William Paulet in command, was obliged to give the Sardinians room, and he was thinking of giving them our General Hospital; at first, we did not credit it, but the story strengthened. We knew the only Sardinian hospital on the Bosphorus was one of huts at Yenikoi, and that long ago when Lord William held the command, he had offered them the one at Abydos, which they declined, as being at so great a distance from the camp; but thoughts and plans were suddenly interrupted by the real news that Sebastopol had fallen. There was no doubt: cannon and flags and information from the embassy confirmed this tale. Graphic accounts from our soldier-friends at camp soon arrived. We insert a letter from one of the sergeants, who had been Sister Anne's ward-master.

> Camp before Sebastopol, 16th Sept., 1855.
> Sister Anne,—Sebastopol has fallen! The enemy is in full retreat! The town is in flames since the 8th. The 2nd and Light Divisions attacked the Malakoff and took it without losing a man; but in attacking the Sedan, the 88th, 55th, and 71st, and other corps of these divisions, suffered severely in trying to take it. Next morning (9th) we were in full possession of this side of the town and part of the north side too. I send you a piece of Russian riband I found in the town (for the French and English were in it plundering by eight o'clock). I have some small oil paintings yet, but the larger articles I gave them to officers of the corps.
> Such beautiful furniture I never saw before in any town, and it is a little dangerous to enter it as yet, for all the houses are filled

with powder. Perhaps we would be ransacking a house and the next one to us would be blown up. Not many hurt in the town after all. Hoping the fall of this terrible fortress will put an end to the war and enable the soldiers of the army to go home to see their friends—the wish of every one of us here, officers, soldiers, and sailors—and hoping you will excuse this scribble,

I remain your most obedient servant,

J. J., 28th Regt.

The news seemed to cheer our men's spirits, who had begun to think that in spite of all they had done and suffered the great object of it all would never be accomplished, and that Sebastopol never would be taken. They illuminated the hospital as well as they could by sticking innumerable pieces of tallow candles (which they either bought or asked the ladies to buy for them) in every pane of every window, and in all other imaginable places; they made candlesticks of common soap, a piece of ingenuity which much amused us.

There were of course grand illuminations all down the Bosphorus, and beautiful fireworks. The ships were all gaily decorated with flags, and the firing of cannon was tremendous.

In the evening the soldiers made a bonfire outside the hospital, into which they threw everything they could lay hands upon, old packing cases, boxes, chests, firewood, planks, and, lastly, a cart belonging to a Greek which happened to be near; they seized upon it, first threw it into the Bosphorus to see if it would swim, and then dragged it out amid shouts of laughter, and threw it on the blazing fire, round which they danced, and sang songs of battle and victory and "*God save the Queen*."

The *commandant* and all the officers stood above both sanctioning and enjoying the festivities. We also looked on at a little distance, accompanied by the whole staff of nurses, who fully entered into the excitement of the scene.

We could not help thinking, however, as we stood listening to the sounds of rejoicing at the glorious victory, of the many aching hearts the news of it would cause in England. Alas! with what sickening suspense would many and many a mother, Sister, wife, and friend watch for the coming lists of killed and wounded, and sadly how to many of them would the fall of the great Sebastopol be the death-blow of their earthly happiness!

True, their loved ones had died a glorious death in the flush of honour and victory, but death, whether on the battlefield or in the silent chamber, is still death and, as we watched the brilliant illuminations that evening on the shores of the Bosphorus, and listened to the repeated hurrahs, we sorrowfully remembered those who would weep tomorrow in England.

The 20th of September was the anniversary of the Alma. The soldiers were anxious to keep the day with honour, and there was a dinner party organised in each hospital: that at the lower consisted of the non-commissioned officers, at the upper the sergeants and orderlies in charge—for this latter plenty of plum-puddings were made in the extra-kitchen, for we liked to do anything to encourage the orderlies.

When they were about to sit down the Reverend Mother spoke to them and begged them to observe temperance and not disgrace themselves. They promised faithfully they would, and when she had retired, they drank her health, with the toast, "*Long may she reign over us*,"; and every man of the party went to bed sober. They were very much pleased with themselves next morning when they found not one was in the guard-room, while at the Barrack Hospitals there were dozens there.

At the Barrack Hospitals we gave our orderlies plum-puddings, but as they were not invited to the non-commissioned officers' dinner, they had them for supper, and enjoyed them very much; but, alas, they did not keep in such good order as their comrades on the hill. Some of the ladies wishing, with perhaps rather more kindness than wisdom, to treat their orderlies on this occasion, gave them a little money, charging them not to drink more than they ought; they promised to remember this, and many kept the promise, but there were a few exceptions.

In No. 3 Upper was an orderly who was always too much inclined to drink; in all other respects he was very valuable, being extremely kind to the patients and attentive to orders. Sister M—— A—— had charge of his ward—when she came next morning to her ward he was missing—she inquired again and again for W——, wanting him to fetch the extras and attend to various other matters, but no one would tell her where her orderly was; there was evidently some mystery connected with him, and at last she very gently but decidedly insisted upon knowing it.

"Where is W——?" said she, "I want him particularly and cannot wait any longer."

"Well, if you please, Sister, he's on the shelf in the linen-press."

She went to the cupboard, and there sure enough he was fast asleep on one of the shelves, where his comrades had laid him, hoping to shield him from punishment. It was so utterly absurd that she had difficulty in looking grave, and thought it best to let the matter pass; but the ladies, on being told of the circumstance, took care not to treat their orderlies in the same way again.

CHAPTER 26

Departure of the Sisters for Balaclava

Immediately after Sebastopol fell, we were told 500 sick, either Russian or British, most likely the former, would arrive. This caused a great commotion—beds were prepared, the new wards looked to, and it was proposed to dismantle the church ward to make room—fortunately it was decided to wait till the sick came before this was done. Every day we looked out for them, and yet they came not; and at last, we found it was only a report, and it began to appear very evident that the hospitals on the Bosphorus would never, in all human likelihood, be filled again (for if the fall of Sebastopol did not bring sick and wounded nothing else would); and the work in the trenches being now at an end the coming winter was not likely to produce the miseries of the last.

Next came the news that General Storks had decided upon giving up the General Hospital to the Sardinians. It was a blow to lose our pretty model hospital just as it was perfect—kitchen stores and wards, each a pattern in its way and all working so well. Still, we felt our regret was rather selfish. There were not fifty patients in this hospital, and for these there was abundance of room in the Barrack Hospital, while our gallant allies, it was said, were in distress.

Next came a letter from Dr. Hall to the Reverend Mother, asking her and her Sisters to come and take the nursing at the General Hospital, Balaclava, which had been under Miss Nightingale's superintendence, and had been attended through the summer by one lady and three or four nurses belonging to Miss Nightingale's staff; but Dr. Hall's letter said that Miss Nightingale had just resigned the charge of General Hospital, Balaclava, into his hands, informing him that her nurses would be withdrawn by the 1st of October. Dr. Hall, therefore, wished the Sisters to come as soon as possible after that day.

He wrote at the same time to our principal medical officer requesting him to make the necessary arrangements for their departure, and apply for passages.

The Reverend Mother asked our superintendent if she could spare her, and though Miss Hutton's regret at losing the Sisters was very great, she said she could not conscientiously hinder them and gave her permission for their departure, and aided in their preparations.

A Catholic chaplain from the camp, Mr. Woolett, came down to escort the Sisters to Balaclava. Mr. Woolett had visited Koulali several times previously. He had been on board the same vessel which brought the ladies and nurses in April, and was therefore welcomed as a friend; his name was also familiar to us being so often mentioned by the patients coming down sick from the camp who spoke with gratitude of the attention he rendered them.

He was indeed one of the many excellent chaplains who distinguished themselves by their devotion to their sacred duties in the camp. An interesting history the deeds they have wrought would make—but most of them are unknown to the world.

In the early spring the number of Catholic chaplains fell far short of that allowed by Government, and the work became very heavy. Mr. Woolett had toiled day and almost night that none should suffer from the deficiency in number. Passages were taken in the *Ottawar*, and preparations were made for the departure of the Sisters. The first week in October was a very busy one, for the General Hospital was to be given over to the Sardinians. Two days before the Sisters left, the patients were moved into Upper Stable Ward (one of the new wards of the Barrack Hospital), stores and furniture were packed up and sent to the purveyor, and numerous packages prepared for the Sisters.

It was necessary they should take a number of things with them, for the accounts from Balaclava were so various. Some said nothing could be had there without paying an enormous price. Mr. Woolett said it was not so, but he had an unusual affection for the camp, and as we feared he made the *best* of things whilst others made the *worst*, it was determined therefore that they should take the middle course.

At length all was ready, and October the 8th was fixed for their departure. Lighters had been ordered to come down from Scutari to take the luggage, but none appeared. At eleven the Sisters could delay no longer, for fear of losing their passage; they ordered as many boxes as possible to be placed in the *caiques*, which were to convey them to the Golden Horn, where the *Ottawar* was lying.

The long train of Sisters descended the hill and entered the barrack-yard. They stopped at the extra store-room to bid farewell to our superintendent and the other ladies. The tears came to our eyes as we parted from them. From first to last the utmost cordiality had subsisted between all the ladies and Sisters, and some of us felt we were parting from tried and warm friends.

Passing down to the quay they were again stopped by the number of patients, orderlies, and soldiers from the detachment, crowding to say goodbye, and shower down a last blessing on the heads of those who had been so long their nurses and comforters. The quay was crowded with soldiers and officers; everyone in the hospital was sorry they were going, for their simple holy lives had won the respect and goodwill of all.

They embarked in *caiques*, and were soon on board the *Ottawar*. Among their fellow passengers was one going to the camp, whose departure all deeply regretted. Mr. Coney, the senior Church of England chaplain, was ordered to the station of St. George's monastery, and to our real sorrow he quitted us. Our only consolation was that he would have a wider field of work in which to do good; very much indeed had he done at Koulali, and among those who differed from him in religion, as well as those who agreed with him, he was universally respected and beloved.

I took my last farewell of the Sisters on board the *Ottawar*. There I met and was kindly greeted by Miss Nightingale, who was also going up in the *Ottawar*, with two nurses, to the Castle Hospital, Balaclava. The Sisters of Mercy, from the General Hospital, Scutari, also here joined their Superioress and the rest of their community, as the whole number were to proceed together to Balaclava.

The General Hospital, Koulali, was closed formally the next day, and the Sardinians were daily expected. Days passed into weeks, and yet no signs of their arrival. The departure of the Sisters made a terrible blank; we could not bear to go near the General Hospital, where we had spent so many happy hours—now gone for ever. General Storks expressed his sorrow at their valuable services being lost to the hospitals in his command.

The medical officers spoke in the highest terms of the assistance they had rendered while under their orders. One of them inquired into the peculiar rules of their order. He had never met with nuns before, and fancied all religious orders were cloistered, of which life he said he did not approve, but thought an active order like this most useful.

Invalids were sent home after the Sisters' departure, so that our numbers diminished more and more, while twice a week as usual a number of men were discharged for duty while none came down from the camp. We had now only one hundred men in the Barrack Hospital, and another one hundred and ten in the Convalescent Hospital, who were not under our care. We began seriously to contemplate the advisability of some of our party returning home, as it was evident that the closing of the General Hospital and the diminution of patients had more than counterbalanced the loss of the Sisters, and our staff was far too large for our present work.

Those who had important duties at home, and who had left them only because they were called out by a great emergency, did not feel justified in remaining when that emergency had passed.

One had almost made up her mind to leave when an alteration in the routine at once caused her and others also finally to decide on returning to England. Dr. Humphrey had for some time past considered that the health of the patients had so amended, and the facility of procuring things from the purveyor's stores was so great, that he thought the old routine of the diet-roll ought again to be revived.

An act of disobedience of one of the hired nurses brought matters to a crisis, and Dr. Humphrey issued general orders to the effect that nothing was to be given except from the diet-rolls. This order came so suddenly that we were dismayed by it. It was issued to all on November 2nd, and carried into effect with military rapidity. The ladies' plans of nursing were upset, and they did not know what to do with themselves, so they assembled in the store-room, looking very blank, and complaining to our superintendent. The lady in charge of the storeroom, who had been thinking of going home, now laughingly declared the matter was settled, for her work was done.

In a few days the ladies saw the reasonableness of Dr. Humphrey's regulation—hospital routine had been infringed upon for many months. The infringement began at a time of distress unknown in the annals of military hospitals; it had been carried on beyond that period, and the time for its discontinuance had arrived.

A regulation once made for a military hospital should not be broken. If it is not sufficient for the wants of the men it should be altered; if it is sufficient it should be obeyed. However, one evident conclusion arose from this change. Some of us must return home, leaving a sufficient staff for the hospital should it ever happen (which was unlikely) to be full again. The numbers then at Koulali exceeded this.

Five of the lady volunteers sent in their resignations to General

Storks. He accepted them in the kindest manner, regretting our intended departure, but agreeing that our decision was a wise one.

The superintendent being among those who resigned another was appointed, who was Sister Anne, the only volunteer lady remaining. There was, however, some rumour of the Barrack Hospital now being emptied of patients and given up to the German Legion, for whom room was wanted. General Storks did not wish to do this, as he thought the landing place at Koulali so convenient for the sick in the rough weather which was expected in the winter, but he had to suspend his decision till he could communicate with the Government at home; he therefore requested our superintendent to remain in office till this point was decided.

The other three ladies and myself were set at liberty, and able to enjoy some of the wonderful sights of the East ere we returned to England. We much regretted that our superintendent could not accompany us, especially as she had never, save on two visits of business to Lady Stratford, left the hospital during her stay in it.

Chapter 27

The Bazaars of Stamboul

Our first visit was to the far-famed bazaars of Stamboul. The contrast of shopping there to shopping in Pera is striking. You hardly ever meet a Frank in Stamboul; none are permitted to reside there.

Disembarking at Galata we traversed the bridge, and on reaching the Stamboul side were assailed by a group of worthies who called themselves interpreters—their knowledge of the English and French languages ranging from twelve to twenty words, but who were able to supply all deficiencies by their abundant use of signs. In an evil hour does an unfortunate traveller engage one of these gentlemen to attend him. The presence of one entails upon you that of a dozen—they declare they are all "brothers"—and they follow you about like a pack of dogs.

They only allow you to buy at the shops they select, and at all these they have an understanding with the shopkeepers by which they get a percentage on all you may happen to buy. They do not allow you to speak; they surround you, and shout in their own languages a mixture of Greek, Turkish and Armenian, till your head fairly swims, and you are willing to buy the article at any price to escape from the noise.

Both Greeks and Turks always talk as loud as we should shout, and jabber and gesticulate so as to make you think they are on the point of proceeding to blows; but they are quite calm in reality all the time. When we grew wiser, and came to Stamboul with our own interpreters, it was a delight to walk through the bazaars. True, they are dark and dirty, narrow, and paved as badly as the streets of Pera, but one could fancy oneself transported back to the days of one's childhood, and that the scenes described in the *Arabian Nights*, to which we listened with rapt attention, were now realised.

Here were the embroidered slippers, pipes, divans, rich stuffs, bright colours, and all the wonders which one's fancy had painted. Here were the jewellers and the charm-makers, and here were Damascus scarves and Broussa silks, and glittering table covers and bags, and tobacco pouches of every shade of colour and richly embroidered, and here at the corners of the streets were the tables of the money-changers. Here instead of counters were the divans whereon the Turk sat quietly and smoked his *chibouque*, and did you wish to make a bargain you sat down also on the divan, and gravely, by means of your interpreter, discussed the subject.

You fix perhaps on a pair of Turkish slippers which the interpreter advises you to give thirty *piastres* (five shillings) for. You say "*hatch grosh?*" (how much?) the Turk informs you it is one hundred *piastres*; the interpreter says "*Mashallah!*" throws up his hands, and laughs scornfully. The Turk does the same. You rise to go and proceed on your way, but are suddenly recalled and told you may have it for the thirty *piastres*.

It has a singular effect to look down the streets of the bazaars and see each long row of divans entirely furnished with one particular article. One street of embroidered slippers, another *fezs*, another bags, another jewellery, another cashmeres, and so on. The extreme brilliance, richness of colour of the Turkish manufactures adds much to the effect. The cashmere bazaar is beautiful. The blue and geranium colours are unequalled in their peculiar richness of colour, while the soft texture of the materials exceeds all European manufactures, which is the reason why the dresses of a group of Turkish women fail to produce the gaudy effect which such a variety of colours would have in England.

They always dress in one colour, but in a group one will be in blue, another in green, another in geranium, another in orange, another in yellow, another in lavender, and the colouring of each is so exquisite that they *en masse* look more like a bed of flowers than anything else.

At times the bazaars are much crowded, and many Turkish, ladies may be seen, for shopping appears to be their great amusement. Turkish carriages filled with ladies occasionally pass through the bazaars, obliging the foot passengers to climb on to the divan to escape being trodden down.

Here and there vendors of lemonade offer refreshing draughts to the weary traveller. Then, again, in small white saucers, is a dainty, somewhat resembling blancmange, which the Turks seem to consider very inviting; then tables and trays full of pistachio nuts, chesnuts, and almond cakes can be found; but if any other refreshment is needed the traveller must wend his way to Pera, for he will not get it in Stamboul.

Sow we come to the *chibouque* bazaar, and find pipes of every variety; the cherry-stick, either rough or polished, or richly painted, the amber mouth-pieces of all sizes—the imitation amber and the commoner kind of pipes. Then there are the shops, in which all sorts of knickknacks are to be bought; the beautiful amber-bead chaplets, the same of red Jerusalem-beads; also, sandal-wood, with its sweet scent. Almost every Turk one meets carries in his hand a chaplet, or string of beads in three divisions—thirty beads in each division, and divided off by larger beads—the whole finished with a long shoot of the same material as the beads.

Then there are the *pastilles*, wrapped in gold leaf, one of which is sometimes put into the *chibouque* to add to the fragrance of the tobacco; the coffee cup-holders, in chased silver or carved wood; the tiny coffee cups themselves of china. The bracelet chains, and little bags made of pressed rose leaves, coloured black. These are the leaves of the roses after the *attar* has been pressed out of them.

Then there is the celebrated *attar* itself, and scents of all kinds, of which our interpreter seemed to think the English were very fond, as he always invited us to buy them, and was much surprised if we refused. Then there are the little boxes of henna and black paint, with which the Turkish women stain their finger-nails and colour their eyebrows and eyelashes; and the "*mastic*," which they constantly chew, in order to add to the whiteness of their teeth.

Next come the large Turkish fans, some made of straw, and the more expensive ones of peacocks' feathers, with a small looking-glass in the centre. The principal amusement of the ladies in the carriages seemed to be surveying themselves in this glass, arranging their *yashmacs*, which were sometimes made of extremely fine transparent muslin, especially when there was a beautiful face underneath. Some of the cheaper fans, made of common feathers or straw, we found very useful in the hospitals during the summer.

Then there is the literary bazaar, where the Turk sits cross-legged, looking very grave and very wise, writing and transcribing Turkish characters, which we did not understand, but were struck with the look of superior intelligence and extreme interest displayed on the faces of those thus engaged.

Next the jewellers' bazaar, of which they seem very proud. They think a great deal of jewellery, at least to judge from the quantity the ladies wear both on their hands and heads. The lower class of women also are seldom seen without a large jewelled ring on their finger, or brooch to fasten their *yashmacs*. Then there is the tobacco, which is so much prized in England, and which is less than half the price, I believe, in Turkey, owing to the high duty to which it is subject in this country.

There are also the sweetmeat shops, principally outside the bazaars, looking very gay with their bright-coloured bon-bons, candied sugar, and white and rose-coloured *arrachle*-comb, which is the principal Turkish sweetmeat, and of which it is reported the *Sultan's* ladies eat so much that he rather complains of the expense. It is a sort of sweet gummy substance, with either pistachio nuts or almonds stuck into it, and it is somewhat expensive. The Turks sell this and the tobacco, and several other things, by the "*ock*," which is about two and a half pounds English weight.

The Turkish weights are different to ours, their pound being about twelve ounces. The currency is chiefly in paper. There are two notes— one ten *piastres*, another twenty. There are also gold and silver pieces, but these are seldom used. Bracelets are made of the Turkish silver or gold coins. The Turks always prefer English money, and in making a bargain inquire whether you will pay in English money.

Passing through the bazaars we soon came to the building called the epitaph of Sultan Mahmoud. It is a circular one, and contains his tomb, of which we only gained a sight by peeping through the windows. The tomb is richly ornamented with sculpture, and beside it we saw an *imaum* in prayer. Within the outer enclosure is a garden, in which is a fountain of water, with iron cups fastened to it, so that all who choose may drink. These fountains are generally found outside in all large mosques, providing water for the poor being considered a religious duty, and a great boon it must be to the poor Turks in the parching heat of summer.

Among the most curious sights of Constantinople are the aqueducts. The first of these is Yere Batan Serai, intended to supply the city with water in case of a siege, as the soil of Constantinople does not produce drinkable water; the water is conveyed to it from Belgrade, or rather the great aqueducts six miles from that town, the arches of which can be seen in the distance from Buyukdere. *Yere Batan Serai*, or the swallowed-up palace, is one of the most remarkable constructions ever known. It would appear that nearly the whole of Constantinople is undermined with it, for none can ever discover its extent; different parts of the roof have fallen in, and three accidents have occurred at quarters of the city miles distant from each other. All these cisterns must have been built in the first two centuries after the foundation of the city. The roof of the mysterious water-palace is supported by marble pillars, each formed of a single block.

Bin Vebir Direg, or cistern of the thousand and one, is the next object of interest. The name implies that the roof is supported by 1,001 columns, but in reality, there are but 336. There were three storeys to this cistern, though but one is now accessible; it has been reckoned that when these three storeys were full, they alone contained sufficient water for the whole number of inhabitants of Constantinople for ten or twelve days. The columns are formed of several blocks, and the marble is much coarser than that of Yere Batan Serai; narrow windows closely grated and built near the roof admit the light. The cistern is entirely filled up. When Signor Fossati was repairing Santa Sophia some years since, the soil taken out was thrown into *Bin Yebir Direg* and the water courses turned off. The immense space thus left vacant is overspread by silk-workers.

Descending a ladder, we found ourselves in this mysterious subterranean palace; wending in and out among the columns were the long lines of silk, which we could just distinguish in the dim light, looking like magic threads; while the strange beings at the works, with their pale faces (for the atmosphere is most unhealthy), their rapid movements at their weaving, and the shrill tones of their voices shrieking to us not to injure their silk, which the hollow echoes repeated, made the scene a most unearthly one.

The air was so stifling that we hastened to quit this horrible place, but before doing so were assailed by a group of the wild, haggard-looking silk-workers catching our clothes and begging vociferously for "*backshish.*" We were indeed thankful to gain the open air.

At a short distance from the *seraglio* a Greek gentleman, who was kindly escorting us, stopped at the door of a large building guarded by sentries; there was a little demur as to our admittance, but the sight of the uniform of an English officer, also of our party, and a little additional *backshish*, as usual carried the day, and the door flew open. Upon entering I started back, for just before me stood a Turk of enormous stature, fierce countenance, and threatening gesture. A burst of laughter from the sentry reassured me, and I discovered the fierce-looking figure before me was made of plaster.

We then entered a large hall, from which four rooms opened, and we found ourselves in a Turkish "Madame Tussaud's." All round these rooms were glass cases, in which were ranged hundreds of plaster or painted wooden figures larger than life. About in the hall these figures were placed in groups; they were mostly arrayed in the warlike costumes worn by the different regiments of the once famous *janissaries*, and were put there by order of Sultan Mahmoud, who after he had succeeded in destroying this formidable body of men was anxious that their dress should be perpetuated.

One specimen of the dress of each regiment was here, and the effect of the many varieties of costume was curious enough. The artist had succeeded admirably in his work, for the various countenances of these gaunt figures gave us a complete idea of the fierce race they were intended to represent.

Besides those of the *janissaries* there was a representation of each minister of state and the principal *imaums*. The turbans of some of the figures were very singular, consisting of rolls of white calico twisted till they were five feet high; others had high felt hats, either square or conical, about four feet high. One case contained very different figures; they were made of wax, and were representations of Circassian or Georgian women, probably some beauties of the *Sultan's harem*. Their soft complexions and beautiful, though unintellectual faces, formed a strong contrast to the ferocious warriors around them.

We were struck by the evidence afforded of the Sultan Mahmoud's bold infraction of the command in the *Koran*, forbidding all human representations. There was something extremely painful in this sight. The figures, though so rude, had a horrible lifelike look: the fierce eyes seemed to glare at one, and it was with a sensation of extreme relief that we quitted the Elbicei Atika.

The *Atmeidan*, or ancient hippodrome lies behind the *seraglio*. Here is all that remains now of ancient Byzantium, the obelisk of Theodosius, and the serpentine column. The last is inscribed with hieroglyphics: it is supposed to be at least 3,000 years old. The serpentine column consisted of three serpents entwined, all of which have lost their heads long ago. It is nearly in ruins, and the base sunk into the earth. Its origin is quite uncertain. Some suppose Constantine caused it to be transported from Delphos, but this is not authenticated.

One great interest will ever attach itself to the great plain of the *Atmeidan*, for here took place the massacre of the *janissaries* by Sultan Mahmoud. For long years the *sultans* of Turkey had groaned under the yoke of these oppressors. The *janissaries* were so powerful a body that they set all laws at defiance, and virtually ruled the empire. The reforms wrought by Sultan Mahmoud gave them such displeasure that endless seditions were fostered by them.

At length an open rebellion burst forth; they overturned their soup-kettles, and threatened to fire the city. (The *janissaries* when marching carried before each regiment a large soup-kettle instead of a standard.) And assembled at their barracks, situated at one end of the *Atmeidan*.

The brave *Sultan* summoned the few troops on whom he could depend, and headed them himself. The battle began. The *janissaries* retreated into their barracks, and there the fight turned into a massacre; for the *Sultan's* troops set fire to the buildings and all were consumed. About 5,000 *janissaries* perished on that day, and the troop was extinct. The *Sultan's* vengeance was not sated till the turban on the tomb of every deceased *janissary* was knocked off, and many of their decapitated monuments are to be seen in the great cemeteries.

Near the *Atmeidan* stands the Mosque of Sultan Achmet. Its chief beauty consists in the colossal proportions of the four columns which support the whole weight of the building. Turkish relics, highly valued by the nation, are kept here, but not exposed to view. Like most mosques, it was without furniture or decorations.

On the last Friday we spent in the East we intended to have seen the dancing *dervishes*, and went to Galata for that purpose; but, to our great disappointment, the Armenian gentleman who had promised to escort us, informed us on our arrival that a fire the previous night had burnt the *Tehle* or *dervishes'* house to the ground. They would not therefore dance until the following Friday; and before that day arrived, we had left the East.

As we could not visit the *dervishes*, we proceeded to the French hospital at Pera. Our kind Armenian friend had procured for us the only two carriages with springs to be hired in Pera. We drove to the hospital, which is distant about two miles from Pera. This building is a very fine one, admirably adapted for an hospital. We proceeded to the apartments occupied by the *Soeurs de la Charité*, twelve of whom are attached to this hospital. By them we were conducted through the wards—they were nearly empty.

Those who were wounded in the assault of Sebastopol had recovered, and from fifteen hundred the numbers had been reduced to five hundred.

We had long been anxious to visit this hospital, having heard much of it from our very first arrival in the East. During the time of distress in our own hospitals it had been spoken of in high terms as possessing all we then so much needed. This was probably the case, but many months had passed, and now certainly we had outstripped our allies in the appearance of our hospital. However, it must be considered that during the summer, while *our* hospitals were empty, *theirs* had been crowded. The wards for both officers and men were inferior in cleanliness and general appearance of comfort to those at Koulali and Scutari, but of the management and routine of the French hospital we had, of course, no means of judging.

From Pera we drove to the castle of the Seven Towers, or the old state prison where captives were immured under charge of the *janissaries*. Even foreign ambassadors were among these prisoners when war was declared against the countries they represented; for the Turks in those days did not think it worthwhile to keep faith with Christians.

Times are changed indeed when the empire would be lost were not Christian blood shed to defend it. An older and sadder history even than theirs still clings to these now ruined walls. Beneath them was fought the last battle between the Ottomans and Greeks; there the Cross fell before the Crescent, and from that victorious battlefield Mahomet II. rode into the city.

The ruins of the Seven Towers had till lately long been deserted and silent, but busy sounds were once more heard among them. One of the numerous French hospitals was erected among the ruins, which are fast falling into utter decay. This hospital consisted entirely of huts, which were neatly built and had every appearance of comfort. The wards were beautifully clean, far more so than the stone ones at Pera. We saw one hut raised on a mound of earth. On entering we found it was the extra diet kitchen, furnished with a charcoal stove and boilers; the flooring being the uncovered ground. Several soldiers were very busy cooking, and a Sister of Charity superintending.

In the centre of this hut was an immense space, boarded round and covered with planks. On inquiry we found it was an old well, into which the *janissaries* were wont to throw some victims of their vengeance. Some of the boards were removed to allow us to look down, and the soldiers took brands from the fire and cast them into it that we might see by the glare, as they descended, the fearful depth, and the water at the bottom; one brief look was quite sufficient, and the boarding was replaced.

At this moment the French principal medical officer of the hospital entered to give some directions to the *Soeur*, and taste the soup, &c., which she was preparing for the patients. We were struck by the extreme courtesy of his manner to her, for although she was evidently not a lady either by birth or education, her office inspired more respect than if she had possessed both. The French doctor spoke courteously to us, expressing his pleasure at our visit to his hospital. Three huts were set apart for the Sisters; use, a fourth formed the chapel. There were at least one hundred huts altogether. They appeared so securely built that we were astonished to hear from *Madame la Supérieure* that the rain came through in torrents, so that in wet weather the inhabitants were obliged to sleep under umbrellas.

The Seven Towers were built on the summit of a hill, and exquisite is the view which lay stretched before the eyes of the poor captives who spent their weary days within their walls—how they must have pined to be beside the blue Bosphorus breathing the free air of heaven!

After leaving the castle we drove about a mile further on, and arrived at the summit of the hill above Bebek, which is so steep that the carriages could not descend without injuring their springs; so, we left them there, walked down the hill, and crossed to Koulali in *caiques*. The drive from Pera to the Seven Towers is one of the few that can be taken in a European carriage, as the ground is tolerably level for some miles, but the country around is very barren and uninteresting.

CHAPTER 28

Visions of the Past

There is one spot in Constantinople to which the heart of the Christian must ever turn with the most intense interest. Old Roman and Byzantine remains, subterranean palaces, records of the ferocious *janissaries*, all fade away into nothingness as we approach the door of

Agia Sophia (the Church of the Eternal Wisdom). This great edifice stands at the north of the *Atmeidan*, on an elevated ridge; the northern end of which ridge reaches to Seraglio Point.

Close by Santa Sophia once stood the great palace of the Caesars, divided from it only by the forum of Augustus, which formed a common entrance to both church and palace. The gardens and terraces of the palace of the Caesars must have extended from the ridge on which Santa Sophia was built to the seashore. We stood before Santa Sophia at the principal entrance through which the *Sultan* had entered on the Beiram. Here we were positively refused admittance.

We then proceeded to a side entrance, and on passing within the porch descended a flight of stone steps and found ourselves in a portico amid a host of *imaums*. A few yards from us was a door covered only with carpet hangings. To our left was another small door, made in the wall, closely locked. Here ensued the usual quarrel with *imaums* about *backshish*.

I paid several visits to Santa Sophia, but shall condense all that I saw and learnt about it in one account. At these different visits we paid various sums for admission; at the time of *Ramazan* it was very high, and there was a great uproar before we gained admittance; we then paid one hundred *piastres* for a large party, at other times we paid less.

At length this knotty point was settled; one of the *imaums* opened the door in the wall and made us follow him, carefully locking it behind him. A winding inclined plane led us up to the women's gallery; in the centre of this are raised some wooden steps, ascending which we obtained a more extensive view of the church.

The first feeling is that of admiration at the vastness of this wonderful building, and not the least part of this wonder is that the whole extent of the dome flashes on one at the first glance. One does not have to wait, as it is said people do, when they enter St. Peter's at Rome, to calculate the vastness; for there, I have heard it is not till you walk under the dome you see it to advantage. Standing on the threshold of Santa Sophia one sees the whole extent of the dome as well as the greater part of the interior at a glance.

Santa Sophia as a mosque possesses neither ornament nor decoration of any kind, save a number of immense green shields engraven in gold, with sentences from the *Koran*, which are hung upon the pillars covering the capitals; a number of silver lamps are also hung around. The *Nimber* and *Mihrab* or desk, from which the *Koran* is read, stands in that part which was once the chancel. Opposite to this a gilded throne for the *Sultan;* an old carpet hangs at the east end, its only value consisting in its having come from Mecca, and this is all.

Great care has the Mussulman taken to hide every token of the former possessors of Santa Sophia; the flooring is covered thickly with matting—plaster has hidden the mosaic walls and roof. A few Turks, both men and women, were prostrating themselves on the matting, and the monotonous howl in which they pray was echoed up to the gallery, sounding almost like the cry of evil spirits. The *imaums* in the gallery eagerly pressed us to buy some little bits of mosaic which they are always pulling down from the walls to sell.

And this was Santa Sophia in 1855, but thought would not rest here. This was no mosque like Sultan Achmet's, which one entered only to admire marble pillars and vast proportions. This was a Christian church, however desecrated. It was once the especial dwelling of the Lord of hosts, and memory carried one away into those far off years to trace the history of Santa Sophia, and treasure up its wondrous annals. We thought of its first building by Constantine, in 326.

Although this building—which was supposed to be of wood—was destroyed by fire, the present church stands on the exact site of the ancient one, and in the gallery parts of the pillars of the first building have been used in constructing .the second, so that all the memories which cling to the church built by Constantine attach themselves to the work of Justinian, and we gazed down from the gallery and tried to forget the present scene and the false worship while the visions of the past rose up before the mind's eye. To follow the whole of that long history would be impossible, but there are some scenes written indelibly upon its pages.

Thought transports one back 1,400 years. The vast church is filled with an eager multitude; the women's gallery is crowded with noble ladies: among them sits the Empress Eudoxia, in all her pomp. The sounds of Christian worship ring through those old walls; bishops, priests, and deacons stand around, and now rises one from amidst their number—a man whose pale face tells the tale of fast and vigil, and how in solitude he learned the secret of that wonderful eloquence which shall make the heart of that great multitude quiver as one man. Yes, there he stands upon the altar steps, a man low in stature but great in soul, the patriarch of Constantinople, St. John Chrysostom.

And now he speaks, and awestruck they all listen to those words of fire. Are they words of burning warning that he is pouring forth, or are they those addresses of ardent love, in which he told them that he would lose his sight for their sakes, because sweeter to him than all the sights of this fair world was the salvation of their souls? (*Life of St. Chrysostom*) and as he pauses there is a stir in the vast assembly. According to the custom of the age their admiration bursts forth—they wave their garments and plumes, lay hands upon their swords and shout, "Worthy the priesthood: thirteenth apostle, Christ hath sent thee." (*Characteristics of Men of Genius.*)

But these sounds of praise—generally liked by the preachers of those days—had no effect on that stern spirit. He knew the world's applause was fleeting, and bids his hearers show, not by words of acclamation but by tears of penitence, that he had touched their hearts, and he judged well. Not long was Santa Sophia to be filled with admiring crowds, not long did the haughty empress listen to his fervid words—truth was not palatable to that luxurious court.

The scene is changed, no longer do they listen within the church and bend before the altar; they who had praised him rose up against him and drove him into exile. He crossed over to Asia, but his foes did not triumph long. A violent earthquake shook the city, and the affrighted people thought it was a judgment upon them for the sin of his banishment. They sent messengers to recall him, the whole city went out to meet him. The Bosphorus was bridged across with boats, and lighted up with torches. Two short months passed by, while he prayed and preached within Santa Sophia's walls, when the storm of persecution recommenced.

A silver statue of the empress was placed before Santa Sophia's doors, and around it the people danced and feasted, and sounds of the wild revelry of a great multitude pierced through the wall and drowned the songs of praise. Chrysostom thundered forth his stern rebuke, though knowing that bitter persecution would be his portion, fearlessly the bishop denounced their impiety, and now the empress was resolved on a lasting vengeance. Santa Sophia's floor was stained with blood, for the emperor's troops came even on Easter eve, the day of all the year of holy calm, to drive the people from the church where St. Chrysostom is ministering.

A few weeks of struggle pass away—when the songs of Whitsuntide should be ringing through the church, there are instead sounds of weeping and mourning. Can we not fancy we see him now before the high altar in Santa Sophia, praying the Eternal Wisdom to direct his steps?

They bring in the sentence of his banishment. No more must he teach the flock, for whose salvation he had so yearned; that tongue whose eloquence the world has never equalled, was to be stilled for ever. Perhaps before his eyes floated some vision of the woe which was to fall over the city, and desecrate his loved cathedral.

Around him gather his bishops, and when he parted from them his last words were, as if in prophecy, "Farewell to the angel of this church." Embracing them with tears, and blessing the deaconesses who flocked around him, and in touching words entreating that they would offer up prayers for their exiled bishop, and then avoiding the attention of the multitude, he went to his doom to wander three years in the wilderness, dragged about by brutal guards—rest at night—clean water to drink, bread to eat were often denied to him whom once in Santa Sophia the people almost worshipped.

No murmur passed the saintly lips—they led him through the scorching heats which poured down their fury on that bald head they led him out in rains till he was drenched in streams of water. At last, the hour of release was at hand; he asks for rest, for he knows death is near; the guards only drag him on more violently than before. But there is a Power stronger than they. At last, they are forced to lay him in a roadside chapel, and there he called for the white garments of his priesthood, and saying in death that which had been his song through life, "*Glory be to God for all things*,'" went to his rest.

Thus died the great Patriarch of Constantinople; his memory is the principal interest which attaches to the former church of Santa Sophia.

In 532 this temple was laid in ruins by fire. Justinian then sat on the throne. He was a great man, and he conceived the mighty ambition to build a church which should excel the temple of Solomon. The foundation of it was laid forty days after the fire. In less than six years his work was completed, and Justinian beholding it, exclaimed, "Solomon, I have conquered thee!"

During the reign of this emperor an earthquake did great damage to the church. Its ravages were, however, perfectly restored, and for 1,300 years, though countless earthquakes have shaken the city, not one has touched Santa Sophia. Against fire Justinian carefully preserved it, for he ordered his builders to employ fire-proof materials; this has been carried out even to the doors and windows—the tracery work of the windows is of stone and the doors either of bronze or covered with it. Some of the windows, it is said, contain panes of the oldest glass ever made, but the date of their insertion is unknown. In the apse of the eastern windows are inner windows of coloured glass, which the Turks allow to remain as a curiosity.

The *imaums* drew our attention to these, and pointed them out with evident pride. The door frames are of bright-coloured marble, except that which was the emperor's entrance-door, and which was of bronze. Over all the doors are large hooks, or rings, as it was customary to suspend hangings or veils before the church door. This is now a universal custom in the Greek churches; the door curtain is always made of some heavy material, with bars of wood placed in it, so that it is difficult to lift. The emperor's entrance-door is adorned with a bas relief, it consists of an arch supported by columns; beneath, is a throne, over which is the Holy Ghost as a dove descending from heaven, holding in the beak the book of the Gospel, having written outside "*I am the door of the sheep.*"

The other doors were not remarkable except those at the south end; these are of planks of timber, four or five times thick, covered with bronze. The ornamental work of the door is so graceful and beautiful that it is supposed to belong to the most brilliant time of Grecian art.

Sculpture was not much thought of in the way of ornament in Santa Sophia, save in the employment of rare and costly marbles, these were brought together by Justinian from every quarter of his vast empire. Whole walls in the interior and the porches were covered with these magnificent materials from floor to cornice; masses of bright colours were arranged in stripes, and bands, and patterns, interspersed with white.

We left the women's gallery and descending the winding passage found ourselves once more in the portico. Another uproar ensued before we were suffered to cross the threshold. We were obliged to take off our shoes, and then the curtain was lifted and, in a moment, we found ourselves on the floor of the far-famed temple. The *coup d'oeil* was marvellous; from arch to arch as one glances up to the stupendous height of the dome—what must it not have been in the days of its glory and beauty!

There have been some fortunate enough within the last few years to have gained some idea of it, for in 1847, the present *Sultan* being alarmed that Santa Sophia was falling to decay, determined on a complete repair, and engaged the services of Signor Fossati, the celebrated Italian architect, by whom it was most successfully accomplished. During this restoration the marble of the floor, the mosaic, and other beauties were uncovered; and the *Sultan* even allowed them to be copied, stipulating only that they should be recovered, as contrary to the law of the *Koran*.

Upon Santa Sophia Justinian and his successors poured every imaginable splendour—the old idol temples were ransacked of their ancient treasures for this purpose—they brought the dark red porphyry from the Temple of the Sun at Rome, and dark green from Thessaly for the columns, while the cornices were of white marble, and on the white they carved the palm leaf in deep relief, covering it with gold. The pillars standing near the emperor's public entrance were carved with four white doves, with passion-flower and cross between; the flooring was all of costly marble; the nave and women's gallery of white and grey, the rest of bright colours, all bordered with verd antique. But the great beauty of all was the mosaic. Walls and roof were covered with it; the whole grounding was of gold, the pictures of saints and angels, groups of flowers, or holy emblems in colours.

Silver mosaic was largely used, and it is believed to have been almost the only church in the world where it was so. The gold and silver mosaic had a peculiar character—it was of glass mosaic, an art of which the Byzantines were masters. On the roof of Santa Sophia thin plates of glass were first fixed with cement, the gold laid upon it, and then covered with a similar plate of glass; it is therefore almost imperishable. Neither the dust of ages nor the whitewashing efforts of the Turks have destroyed its brilliancy.

The most splendid mosaic in the church is that over the emperor's entrance—the representation of the Agia Sophia himself. He is enthroned in glory, His robes are of white and gold, His right hand lifted up as if in the act of speaking; in the left the gospels, on which is written "*I am the light of the world.*" At His feet is prostrated the emperor, clad in his diadem and regal robes, of blue, red, and gold, in the act meant to represent a vassal doing homage to his liege lord. This is supposed to be Justinian himself. On each side of our Lord are medallions of the Mother of God and the archangel Michael.

On the roof of the women's gallery is a representation of the Day of Pentecost. On the west end are figures of the Blessed Virgin, St. Peter, and St. Paul. These are not in good preservation, for the figure of the Holy Child, which was placed with His Mother, is gone—only the crown of glory left. Around this picture is a rainbow.

On the walls are numbers of pictures of bishops and martyrs, and also of six lesser and two greater prophets. Isaiah is holding a scroll with the words—"*A virgin shall conceive and bear a child;*" and with his right hand he points to the sanctuary. There are also the cherubims with their six wings, and other pictures in profusion. The centre picture of the dome is supposed to have been Christ as the Judge of the world, but it is gone.

The rood screen had twelve columns and three doors. Over it stood an archangel with gleaming sword to guard the holy place. The covering and ornaments of the altar were all of gold. The ciborium with silver pillars and veil of rich embroidery; on it hovered the dove, typical of the Holy Ghost.

The holy vessels themselves were one blaze of precious stones. When one reads and ponders over the account of all the splendour of this church, which surely must have been the glory of Christendom, we enter into the feelings of its old historian, who said—"When one once puts a foot in Santa Sophia one desires never to depart from it."

Again, the vision of those old times floats before our sight. One stands in Santa Sophia upon that marble floor, under the shade of that great dome, the candelabra and crowns of light shed their rays on gold and silver, and pictured forms; forth comes the long procession, the many bishops, the sixty priests, the hundred deacons, and other officers, altogether four hundred and twenty-five who served this church—they come to adore the Eternal Wisdom.

****

Besides this large number were 100 door-keepers. It is, however, recorded in the old histories of Santa Sophia, that its clergy served three other churches—the church of the Mother of God, that of the Martyr Theodore, and also that of St. Irene.

****

Anthems soaring loud;
Incense curled up and wreathed on high a cloud;
And all tongues choired adoring cup and host—
Glory to Father, Son, and Holy Ghost. (Moile)

But those days have long since passed; the glory of Santa Sophia was perchance too much for this poor earth—it did not linger long. The church of Constantinople was rent, Chrysostom's prophecy was fulfilled—the angel departed from it.

Storms and dissensions shake the city, the sound of woe is in the air; beneath the Seven Towers the Greeks resist the invaders. In a side chapel, near the women's gallery, in Santa Sophia, an old priest is saying mass; they bring him news that all is lost. He believes them not.

At last, the sound of horses' hoofs is heard, Mahomet II., flushed with victory, rides into Santa Sophia, and, dashing his hand, stained with Christian blood, upon the walls, proclaims its fall.

The old priest pauses. The Turks rush upon him, but the wall of the chapel opening he passes in carrying the holy vessels. They tried to break down the wall, but no power could move a stone. The Greeks aver that occasionally through the walls come faint sounds of psalmody, and when at length the time of their captivity shall be past, and Santa Sophia be restored to God's service, the wall shall re-open of itself, the priest who is now sleeping and chanting in his sleep—shall come forth and finish the interrupted mass. Thus runs the old legend.

As we once more looked around and realised the sad knowledge that the Mussulman desecrated the holy walls of Santa Sophia, earnest was the prayer we silently breathed that God would once more come to His temple, and that the wonderful events of the last few years might be instrumental in paving the way for the restoration of this beautiful cathedral to its former holy purposes. We prayed the time might hasten on when the white robes shall gleam as of old, the floor shall be covered with worshippers among the faithful, and those old walls which have seen Emperors, *Sultans*, and dynasties flourish and decay through so many centuries shall again re-echo with the song of praise,—*Te Deum laudamus*.

Near Santa Sophia stands the old church of St. Irene, built by Justinian; razed to the ground, like Santa Sophia, by fire, it was restored by Justinian. It was served by the clergy of Santa Sophia, and shared its title of patriarchal. It was destroyed by an earthquake in the eighth century, and does not seem to have been restored to its ancient beauty. It is now used by the Turks as a store-house for weapons, and its ecclesiastical remains can only be conjectured. Whatever were its beauties they have now disappeared, but it would seem to have been built upon the plan of Santa Sophia. In the hall, or portico, are deposited some ancient remains of art.

The exterior of Santa Sophia presents nothing worthy of remark; it would appear originally to have had little ornament bestowed upon it, and under the Turkish rule has lost all. It is disfigured by four minarets, marking its unhallowed use, and all round the church are thrown large buttresses. On the western side is an outer court built of brick, but ornamented internally with marble and mosaic work; in the centre of this stood a stone vase for water. This court is now occupied by the dwellings of the *imaums*, which are built in among the old columns and walls. In place of the ancient holy water vase is the fountain for the Turkish ablutions.

The old baptistery stood at the south-west angle of the church; it was octagonal, with eight windows and a vaulted roof. It was first converted by the Turks into a storeroom for oil, and then at the death of Sultan Mustapha was made his tomb; there also his brother was buried. It is still used as the tomb of the *Sultans*, and its memory as the Christian baptistery was utterly lost till Monsieur Salzenberg, in his researches, rescued it from oblivion.

****

In the account of the details of Santa Sophia, I have drawn somewhat largely from the work of the learned Monsieur Salzenberg, Alt Christliche Bandenkmale von Constantinople, feeling sure that as this valuable work is difficult of access in England any information from it would be acceptable, more especially as Monsieur Salzenberg enjoyed opportunities of pursuing his researches in Santa Sophia which will probably during the period of its restoration by Signor Fossati again be afforded in our generation.

****

On the south of Santa Sophia also stood the oratory of St. John the Baptist; this was built previous to the time of Justinian.

CHAPTER 29

Traces of the Knights of Malta

From the time the Sisters of Mercy left us we looked anxiously for letters, and took the deepest interest in their affairs. Everyone who came down from Balaclava was eagerly questioned concerning them and their work, and all spoke of their exertions in the highest terms.

On their arrival at Balaclava, they were lodged in huts built of planks, through the chinks of which the winds whistled cheerlessly. The hospital consisted partly of huts, partly of a stone building. Many civilians were nursed in these huts, men from the transport corps, muleteers, &c., who did not receive even the attention paid to the soldiers.

The huts in which the Sisters lived were so bare and unfurnished that they looked like Indian wigwams, but every hardship seemed but to increase the good Sisters' cheerful zeal, they were so delighted at having plenty of work. They found the character of the work very different from that at Koulali, from patients coming in at all hours, and in a state of acute disease. Cholera prevailed to some extent in October;

the Sisters immediately began night work, and partly owing to the incessant watching many cholera patients recovered.

They had not been many weeks at Balaclava when a sad trial befell them: this was the death of one of the Sisters, the first of their community whom they had lost. After one day's illness with cholera Sister Winifred departed; her death was very peaceful, her Sisters knelt around her bed while the priest recited the prayers for the agonising; they changed into a requiem, and that was the first token to those who watched that the spirit had fled.

Next day, a Sunday afternoon, they bore her to her grave; for this a craggy spot on the hills in view of the huts where the Sisters lived was selected. Priests bearing the cross and chanting led the procession; the coffin was carried by the soldiers for whose sake she had been content to die; the long train of Sisters in white cloaks and bearing tapers followed. Many other people joined them to testify their respect, and so they laid her body in its last resting-place on earth.

The sorrow of the Sisters for their loss did not abate their zeal. One and all were only more anxious rightly to fulfil their appointed work. As time passed on, we heard of the improvements they effected. The orderlies at Balaclava had been a troublesome set, unaccustomed to habits of cleanliness and order; reforms were now introduced and carried out: encouragement from the Sisters and their gentle manners did much more good in teaching the orderlies than all the blame they had previously received.

Just at this time the corps of civil orderlies, reported to be already trained to undertake nursing arrived from England. They landed at Scutari and were soon dispersed among the other hospitals. They all wore a uniform dress of blue smocks, and were pronounced by the soldiers to be "a set of butchers."

The patients did not at all like losing their comrades for orderlies, and I do not think the first few weeks' experience of the "blues" could have been very gratifying to their feelings. I had no personal experience of them, but from what I was told, I fear intemperance prevailed among this corps of orderlies quite as much as among the military ones, and that it was quite as much trouble to train them to their work. At Balaclava the Sisters appeared to encounter a repetition of our great discomforts at Koulali—want of "Etnas," saucepans, &c.

They often regretted their nice kitchen at Koulali, but in course of time their patient perseverance overcame all difficulties, and at Balaclava there is now an extra-diet kitchen and storeroom which rival those of the model hospital.

More comfortable huts have been erected for the Sisters, which they speak of as delightful habitations; and though the winter's cold must have been intense, complaints of the unavoidable hardships never came. When we left the East our last accounts of the Sisters were most satisfactory, their improvements all progressing as well as they could wish. It was pleasing to see the strong interest and affection which continued to be expressed for them after their departure by all at Koulali, and this quite as much so by those who differed from as by those who agreed with them in religion; for all appreciated the gentle courtesy displayed by them to everyone as well as their devotion to their work.

Many asked from whence they had come, and how they had learnt their experience in hospital work. On enquiry we found that their order was a modern one, founded by an Irish lady, a Miss Macaulay, in the year 1831. This order in some respects resembles that of the *Soeurs de la Charité*, but differs from it in others; namely, that its members after passing through a two-and-a-half years' noviciate take perpetual vows. The objects of charity to which the Sisters of Mercy devote themselves are threefold—the education of the poor, visiting the sick, the protection of servants out of place; to these are added others as circumstances require, especially that of the care of hospitals.

In Dublin this work is carried on, and an hospital to be placed under the care of the Sisters is now in the course of erection. This order, founded in Dublin, rapidly extended into many parts of Ireland, and into England and Scotland; from thence it has spread to Australia, New Zealand, America, and California, and a foundation is now just being about to be laid in Buenos Ayres.

It was at last decided that Koulali barracks were to be retained for the present as a British hospital. General Storks therefore appointed Sister Anne as lady-superintendent.

The general offered us passages in the *Hydaspes*, a vessel belonging to the General Screw Steam Company, and then in the employ of the government and laden with shot and shell. She had for some days been lying off Koulali to coal.

The kindness of all around was very great. The men expressed great sorrow at our leaving and were of course very vexed at the alteration in the hospital routine which was the immediate cause of our departure. When it first took place, they thought it must be a great grief to us not to be giving so many "extras," and one day, on going into No. 3 ward, Miss —— found a sheet of paper laid on the table in her ward-room, with some pencilled lines roughly inscribed on it, which were the following—

Though troubles spring not from the dust
Nor sorrows from the ground,
Yet ills on ills, by Heaven's decree,
In man's estate are found, &c.

This piece of sympathy with a grief, which in reality had no existence, was of course a great amusement to us. The lady who received it, brought it home at dinner time, and it was of course welcomed with a peal of laughter. One of the last amusing incidents that varied our hospital days was the visit of a French *Soeur de la Charité*. After passing through the hospital wards, (at the good arrangement and manifold comforts of which she expressed great surprise and admiration) we were passing through the main entrance, and the sentry happened to be a Highlander. I was passing quietly on when my companion suddenly stopped and regarded the Highlander with a look of astonishment.

"*Ah! qui est-ce qui cet homme là?*"

I answered that he was a Scotch soldier.

"*Ah! que c'est drôle. Je n'ai jamais vu un costume si bizarre!*"

She then approached the soldier and looked with great curiosity at his dress. He was delighted at the sensation he made, and showed off his accoutrements with pride, "so sorry" he hadn't his dirk on to show the lady; the pouch, however, received such a share of admiration as ought to have satisfied him.

Dr. Humphrey wrote a letter expressing his thanks for our services, and there was not one from whom we did not receive good wishes. The *Hydaspes* sailed on the 22nd of November; our preparations for departure were quickly made, and our farewells said.

We went on board about four in the afternoon, and we could have started immediately, but the captain was waiting for the Duke of Newcastle, who did not arrive for some hours afterwards, and so the moon rose before the *Hydaspes* heaved anchor. Between our ship and the shore lay a large coal barge; over this one or two of the soldiers chose to climb, that they might say a last "goodbye." A group of them stood on the shore and cheered us on.

The moonlight lit up every familiar spot, as we gave a farewell look to dear Koulali, with which pleasant memories must ever linger. It was some great Turkish *fête*, and the Bosphorus was brightly illuminated as we passed down it.

It would be a needless repetition to describe our route as far as Malta. We found a most delightful change in being on board an English vessel instead of the little crowded French steamer in which we came. The *Hydaspes* is a beautiful ship; it was such a pleasure to walk on her broad smooth decks, and our cabins and the saloon were most comfortable. We received much kindness from all, and especially from Captain Baker, who did everything in his power to make the voyage pleasant to us.

The weather was favourable till we reached Malta, with the exception of one night, in which a gale arose and the cargo of shell was in some way loosened and caused the vessel to roll sadly.

November 27th.—We anchored at the quarantine harbour, Malta, and next day we went into the grand harbour. We remained a week at Malta; the captain's orders being to discharge the cargo of shot and shell there.

The two principal harbours are divided by an oblong peninsula on which is built a castle. Malta is strongly fortified in every direction; these fortifications were built by the knights of St. John, who were masters of it 273 years. The improvements wrought by them were very great, for when Charles V. had offered it to them its barrenness made them hesitate in accepting the gift, while now its means of defence and cultivation are remarkable.

On each side of the harbour is a fortified town; the capital of the island is La Valetta, called after its founder, John of Valetta, a grand master. The town opposite Valetta sustained a severe siege in 1565 from the Turks, but they were completely repulsed, and the town was named Citta Vittoriosa. Valetta, even after all the sights we had seen, was quite new to us; the long flights of steps, the white *stradas*, tall white houses, and innumerable churches were a complete contrast to the East. The great interest, however, attached to Malta, consists in the fact of its being the "island called Melita," which received St. Paul after his shipwreck.

The dress of the Maltese women is very peculiar—it is entirely black; the upper and middle classes wear black silk, and their head-dress is called a *faldette*; it is a large piece of silk made exactly in the shape of an apron, but one side stiffened with whalebone; this is thrown over the head and shoulders, and held by the hand. The very poor women have their dress and *faldette* of coarse material, but always black, and the *faldette* is universal.

Indoors the Maltese ladies wear colours. It is said that the black dress is worn in discharge of a vow made in time of famine or plague that they should wear black for two hundred years, and that, this period being nearly past, they think of changing it; but we hoped it was not true, for it would be a pity indeed that this national and excessively picturesque dress should be laid aside.

Valetta is full of traces of its former governors, the knights. Countless churches built by them, the palace of the Grand Master, the hospital, museum, and public library, all bear witness to their skill and industry; and, when one remembers that they held the island on the condition that they would sustain a perpetual war against the Turks and *corsairs*, one wonders how they found any time and money to spend at home.

The great monument of them labours in Valetta is the church of St. John the Baptist. This saint was the patron of the order. Their original name was Hospitalliers of St. John of Jerusalem, at which city they were founded in 1100. They served hospitals, but considered their duty also called them to fight against the *infidels*. They took an active part in the Crusades. It was not till they had wrested the island of Rhodes from the Saracens in 1308 that they assumed the title of Knights. They were then called Knights of Rhodes till they lost that possession in 1522, and, soon after coming to Malta, were named Knights of Malta.

We were disappointed with the exterior of St. John's church, but on our entrance were fully satisfied. What must it have been in the days of old, when all the colouring and gilding on the walls and the *frescoes* on the roof were fresh, and the choir was filled with the knights in their robes, and their golden cross enamelled in white, with its eight points, in token of the eight beatitudes, and their glittering armour, and when their full chorus rang out gloriously the vesper psalms? Now the beauty has faded, and a few priests and boys chant instead of that mighty peal of praise.

The flooring of St. John's is said to be perfectly unique. It is mosaic, each slab forming a monument to a Knight of St. John. There are 400 of these. At the east end of the church is a large sculpture of the baptism of our Lord. The figure of St. John Baptist is very good. The immense marble pillars are magnificent. The roof is *fresco*, representing scenes in the life of St. John.

In the side aisles are a number of little chapels; in the south aisle is the chapel of the Blessed Sacrament. This chapel is enclosed by chased silver gates of great beauty; it is hung with red silk, and the lights are so well arranged that a soft roseate glow is thrown upon the silver gates and the altar, having an exceedingly lovely effect. Opposite this chapel, in the north aisle, is the Lady Chapel, which was once enclosed by golden gates, but they were carried away by Napoleon. The chapel is very small, and of no remarkable beauty.

At one side of the Lady Chapel is a flight of steps, descending which we reach the chapel containing the tombs of the Grand Masters. There is an altar here, but it is evidently disused. Here in different niches are the sculptured forms of some of the most celebrated Grand Masters of the Order, brass plates and inscriptions to others covering the floor. The principal tombs are of such as distinguished themselves particularly during their government of this island. Here lie all the earthly remains of those "Champions of the Cross," before whose dauntless valour the Saracen so often trembled, and yet who still bore the lowly title of Master of the Hospital of St. John, and Guardian of the poor of our Saviour Jesus Christ.

Wonderful is the history of this grand order, and most remarkable is it that its destruction should have been brought about by treachery. What Solyman could not effect by arms, Bonaparte accomplished with ciphered letters, and from that hour the order was virtually extinct; for though its members, scattered in various parts, lived on for many years, its spirit was gone. They had proved traitors to their island and their oaths, and thus the order crumbled away.

Leaving this chapel, and proceeding down the north aisle, we entered a number of small chapels, called respectively the English, French, Italian, and German. In the French is a large recumbent figure of a brother of Louis Philippe, a very good piece of sculpture. In the English chapel the altar-piece is St. Michael casting out the dragon. We wondered whether this or the one in the Bridgewater Gallery is the original, for the picture is exactly the same, only that the one in St. John's is not in such good preservation as Lord Ellesmere's property.

In the south aisle, nearly at the end of the church is a very large chapel, which the guide said was the oratory, and probably was some chapel used by the knights for their private devotions; now it is disused. The altar of coloured marble was well worth notice. Some of the paintings were also good, but a marble head of St. John the Baptist, kept under a glass case, was a most beautiful piece of sculpture.

We visited St. John's daily as long as we stayed in Malta, and often spent hours, finding out new beauties at every turn. Valetta possesses a great number of churches, most of them raised by the knights, others belonging to religious orders, of whom there are a great many. Numerous as the churches were, they all seemed well attended. In the morning when service was going on they were thronged; in the after part of the day, as often as the explorer entered any of the churches, scattered figures here and there in their picturesque black dress were always to be seen, apparently rapt in prayer.

Sometimes when the church looked quite empty, and we went groping through the side aisles trying by the failing light to discover the merits of paintings or architecture, behind some large pillar one was sure to stumble upon a Maltese woman, looking so like a statue in black marble one could hardly believe she was not one. We visited the cathedral church of St, Paul's, which is very inferior to St. John's. The church of the Dominicans is a fine one. When we entered it the long line of monks in their white habits were chanting vespers in full choir without music.

We also went to the church of San Publilus, who is said by tradition to have been St. Paul's first convert in the isle. There is nothing remarkable in San Publilus but the fine site on which it stands; before it is a large square paved with stones. We were told that this square presented an extraordinary scene once. There had been a drought in Malta for two years, and the Maltese women, after fasting and praying for a week, walked in procession to San Publilus and knelt in the square. The spectators assured us that the whole square filled with figures in black presented a most singular spectacle. The women chanted the *Miserere*. Before the spectators had time to reach home the rain descended in torrents.

We stayed nearly a week at Malta, and had time to see all the curiosities of the island. We drove one day to Citta Vecchia. This town was the ancient capital of Malta before the Knights of St. John held the island. It is still a bishop's See, and contains a cathedral and several convents. We visited the former, but found nothing worthy of note. At Citta Vecchia stands the church of St. Paul, and also the cave. Tradition says it is the one in which the apostle lodged after his shipwreck, where he kindled the fire, and where the viper fastened on his hand.

A priest conducted us into the cave; it was so dark we could not see our way down the rugged flight of steps, but on arriving at the foot of them we did not want any other light than that which is well contrived by a chink in the wall. This soft, subdued light falls on the marble figure of St. Paul, one of the most beautiful sculptures we ever beheld. He is extending the right hand, evidently to show it is unhurt, and the expression of the face is celestial. The spirit of self-sacrifice which characterised the great apostle is written in every line. One of our party remarked, one could almost fancy that the lips would move and say, "*I have imparted unto you my own self also.*"

From the cave we went through the catacombs, from whence it is said there is a subterranean passage to Valetta (a distance of six miles). These catacombs are very extensive and form a perfect labyrinth. As far as we could understand our guide, who spoke very imperfect English, we learnt they were built by the Saracens; and that they were erected long after St. Paul's visit to Malta.

Another day we drove to San Antonio, the governor's palace, and greatly enjoyed our walk round the gardens; the orange trees were loaded with fruit, and many lovely flowers were in bloom. It seemed the only place in Malta where green trees could be seen or cool shade found. The absence of green is a great drawback to Malta; for miles the white houses and the blue sea are the only objects, and the eye gets wearied with the continual glare.

At Valetta we visited the public library and museum; some curiosities and books were there placed by the knights. There were a good many students in the library poring over some ponderous tomes. The librarian could speak broken English, and was very civil in showing all his wonders. He showed us a broken lamp in the shape of a fish, which he said had come out of the catacombs at Rome, and had been used by the early Christians. In the library we were delighted by some illuminated MSS. of great age, but yet in perfect preservation.

Another time we visited some ancient ruins which are supposed to be those of a Phoenician city; but these remains are so few as to be hardly interesting. Malta was first taken by the Phoenicians, who expelled its original inhabitants the Phocians. Returning from these ruins, through a village about two miles from Valetta, our carriage was stopped for half-an-hour by a procession passing through the principal street carrying a large figure of St. Andrew (it was his fete). As the procession reached the church a number of tiny cannons were fired, which seemed to delight the populace. We had not time to do more than look into the church, which was crowded. Around the altar stood a large number of men In the dresses of the various confraternities, who had carried the figure, and who now held lighted tapers.

The body of the church was one dense mass of women, whose

dress being, as before described, entirely black, with the graceful *faldette*, had a striking effect.

Outside the church were many more women and men all kneeling on the ground and seeming rapt in devotion. As soon as the cannon were fired, we were allowed to proceed on our way. The shops in Malta are very attractive, especially those hung with the Maltese lace, and others adorned with jewellery; the Maltese crosses in gold or silver filigree work are extremely pretty.

Quantities of jewellery are displayed in Valetta, and apparently much prized by the ladies, who do not consider gold watches, chains, bracelets, and rings inconsistent with their sombre garb. We visited the Military Hospital, which is situated near the sea. The building was erected by the knights, and is a large and commodious one. Some of the wards are of great extent. It seemed well arranged, but the medical officers told us that, though standing apparently in so good a situation, in reality it is one of the worst that can be conceived—being damp and unhealthy.

The Malta Hospital is a regimental one, conducted on its routine, and therefore not supposed to contain many serious cases, but the surgeons told us that they had had a great deal of sickness since the war broke out, and one did not wonder at this when we saw the troops of young recruits from England who thronged the *stradas* of Valetta, who were such *little boys*, that how they managed to be of the right height we could not think—no wonder they soon fell sick in a foreign country.

There was a review at Valetta one day in honour, I suppose, of the Duke of Newcastle, who had left the *Hydaspes* on her arrival at Malta, and, after paying the governor a short visit, returned to England by the overland route. The review took place in a large square, and was a very pretty sight, though it made us rather melancholy to see all the brave soldiers who were on their way to battle, and perhaps death. Sometimes, though, when walking in the *stradas*, we could hardly avoid a smile at the pride with which the boy soldiers, both privates and officers, walked about in their new uniforms, and we thought how very dim their beauty would become after a few weeks' roughing it in the East.

December 2nd, we sailed from Malta, and on the 10th anchored off Gibraltar. We saw the magnificent fortress under a most favourable aspect, for the last three weeks before our arrival had brought incessant rain, so that Gibraltar was covered with verdure where generally the rock is very arid and bare. We went on shore and climbed up the steep hill to the galleries of the fortifications. These are built in the solid rock.

The stone through which they are cut is so humid that in wet weather it drops with water, thus we found ourselves in a perfect shower of rain, and so put up our umbrellas, and waded through it. We reached St. George's Hall, which is a large space, with a good many cannons ranged round. All along the gallery are portholes, in which are cannon.

From these fortifications we looked down on the sea, the distant mountains of Africa, the town of Gibraltar, and the neutral ground, which, from the rainy weather, was quite a swamp. On one end of this ground stand the English sentries, on the opposite the Spanish. Descending from the fortifications we passed an old Moorish tower, built when the Moors held possession of Spain.

The rain began to fall in torrents, we were tossed about in the boat which conveyed us back to the *Hydaspes*, and were very well pleased to hear we were not to leave harbour that night. Early next morning we were once more on our way. We encountered very rough weather, the screw could not work in so rough a sea, so we were under sail for several days, and were driven out of our course, never entering the Bay of Biscay at all. For several days the weather was so rough we could not stir from our berths.

An attempt to cross the cabin was quite dangerous. We again congratulated ourselves that we were on board so good a ship as the *Hydaspes*; which bravely withstood the storm.

One night the gale was so strong that a sailor was blown overboard, and the sea ran so high that all attempt to save him was useless. At length fine weather returned, the screw was put in motion, and we neared the end of our voyage.

On December the 16th we were called on deck late in the evening to see the Start Light, the first glimpse of Old England. On December the 17th the *Hydaspes* cast anchor off Spithead, and in a few hours more, with very thankful hearts, we were safely at home. One short year only had passed since I left it, but the events of many had been crowded into it.

Here my narrative might end, but that I feel sure my readers will be interested in knowing the fate of those left behind, and especially whether Koulali Hospital continued in its former occupation.

Chapter 30

Accounts from Balaclava

After our departure the fate of Koulali was decided. Sister Anne found the remaining staff of five ladies and ten nurses more than sufficient for the work of the hospital under its present regulations. All went on very smoothly for about a fortnight, the only difference being that the Turkish barracks were given over to the mounted Sappers and Miners, which added greatly to the bustle of the scene—the once quiet road to the Ladies' Home being now thronged with men, horses, and wagons.

During this period a large portion of the German Legion had been sent to Scutari barracks, where in a few days the cholera broke out, numbers dying daily; the troops were immediately marched out and encamped about three miles from Scutari, where they remained ten days.

When the wet weather commenced, it was considered absolutely necessary they should have better protection than a tent, and accordingly on the 4th of December the purveyor-in-chief rode over to Koulali from Scutari with an order from General Storks for the handing over of the Barrack Hospital at Koulali to the German Legion, and the removal of the greater part of the British sick to Scutari, retaining only the Convalescent Hospital for the use of those patients who were unable to be moved at present, and these also, on their recovery, were to join the rest at Scutari, it being intended for the future to keep up the Convalescent Ward for those patients only who should be put on shore there, when it was impossible to land them at Scutari, which was often a difficult matter to accomplish during the winter.

Three medical men were to remain in charge of this hospital, and, the services of ladies and nurses being of course no longer needed at Koulali, General Storks intimated that Miss Nightingale would make arrangements with Sister Anne about engaging those ladies and nurses who might feel inclined to accept her (Miss Nightingale's) rules and wish to join her staff at Scutari in preference to returning to England. This was accordingly settled in the course of the day.

Sister Anne also sent a messenger immediately to the embassy at Therapia, informing Lady Stratford of the sudden changes in the hospital. A violent storm, however, which came on that evening made it impracticable for Lady Stratford to visit Koulali before the final closing of the hospital. Dr. Freeth, the English chaplain, took advantage of a lull in the storm to visit the embassy and explain matters to her ladyship, who sent word by him that she fully intended coming to Koulali the next day; but the storm recommencing her intention was frustrated. The *caidjees* were obliged to land Dr. Freeth at a village a short distance from Koulali, where the party at the Home were anxiously looking out for his return, fearing that from the violence of the storm he might be in danger.

As it was important the Germans should come to Koulali immediately, the bustle and confusion in the hospital were very great. Everything had to be packed up and removed to Scutari. The dismantling of the linen stores was rather provoking, they had been so neatly arranged and completely filled up with everything that was necessary for the men's comfort and convenience. It was half laughable and half annoying to see the "fatigue party" tumbling down the things to take them to the purveyor's stores.

Sister Anne superintended the packing up of the church furniture and fittings, all of which were free gifts from friends in England. She was one of those who had taken great interest in their arrangement, and it was painful to her and others also to see their once neat little church dismantled in a few minutes.

Then came the packing up of the ladies' free-gift store, and this was no little trouble and labour. One of the officers informed Sister Anne that Captain Macdonald wished to have the key of the ladies' store that same evening; she replied that was quite impossible, and that it was unreasonable to expect that everything could be done in a moment. The officer expressed his regret at being obliged to hurry her so much, but begged her to remember that he was "not one of the kickers, but one of the kicked," as he was himself obliged to turn out, as well as the rest of the British officers, to make way for the German ones, the general's orders on the subject being urgent.

Mr. Robertson coming up at this moment, and Sister Anne explaining the difficulty to him, he immediately assured her that the general had no wish whatever that she or any of the party should be annoyed or flurried, and that the key must be waited for till it could be conveniently given up.

About eight o'clock the storm before alluded to commenced, and it was described as one of the most magnificent sights ever witnessed; the lightning was brilliant beyond conception; the night had become suddenly dark, but, as flash followed flash, not only the Bosphorus, but objects on the European coast also, were distinctly visible. The light itself was of a peculiar dark crimson colour, at times fringed with purple, and everything at times became as distinct as by the light of day.

Notwithstanding the beauty of the scene, however, it was impossible to help looking with much anxiety on the Bosphorus raging in its most stormy mood, remembering that Miss Nightingale, who had been at Koulali making arrangements with the ladies, was at that moment on its waves in a small *caique*, as it was impossible she could have reached home ere the storm began, and it certainly is anything but a safe position to be on the Bosphorus in a *caique* even when the water is far less agitated than it was at that time. They heard next day that the storm met her halfway to Scutari, but that she arrived in perfect safety, though completely drenched, for the rain descended in sheets of water.

The next day the packing continued, as it was hoped in a day or two to leave the Home, which was on their departure to be converted into quarters for the British officers still remaining at Koulali; but the Bosphorus continued to rage so violently that no boat, lighter, or even steamer could come from Scutari, and the goods sent there in a lighter on the Thursday before were two days before they could land their contents. A report reached the Home that one steamer bound for Koulali was wrecked on the way. The road to Scutari was almost equally impracticable. It was difficult for a rider to accomplish the journey, much less a vehicle of any kind.

In the meanwhile, what was to become of the British officers, who, by the arrival of the Germans, were now turned out of house and home? Sister Anne at once offered them some of the apartments at the Home, reserving as few as possible for her staff off ladies and nurses. This offer was gratefully accepted, and accordingly Dr. Freeth, the English chaplain, Father O'Dyer, the Catholic one, Dr. Humphrey, the principal medical officer, Major Heaton, the *commandant*, and two or three of the other medical officers, took up their abode in our once quiet little Home, and no doubt the scene was amusing enough.

The whole party dined together, and as the storm lasted the whole of the next week, and the work of the hospital was over, they were somewhat dependent on each other for amusement. Dr. and Mrs. Tice also joined the party, and all did their best to contribute to the general comfort, and to make the best of circumstances which were unavoidable. The time passed pleasantly enough. One of the party had a bagatelle board, and thus helped to while away the idle hours.

At length after ten days' duration the storm ceased, and the sun shone out with really summer-like splendour. The next morning Captain Macdonald sent a steamer to convey the ladies and nurses to Scutari. Sister Anne returned to England in the *Cambria*, under the kind escort of Lord and Lady Napier. Some of the other ladies and nurses also returned in the course of a week or two, a few remaining with Miss Nightingale at Scutari.

From Balaclava favourable accounts continue to be received. The Sisters bravely withstand the rigour of a Crimean winter; looking on the bright side of everything they go cheerfully on working for God, and trusting all else to Him. But since we have been safe in our English homes, many a thought has travelled to those parts in which, amidst cold and rain, far severer than any we experience in England, the Sisters dwell.

The rumours of peace were joyful news to us, bringing with them hopes that ere long, their work done, the Sisters also may return to then peaceful convent homes; but while we were rejoicing over these thoughts the news reached us that one more had already finished all earthly labour, and had gained the shore of everlasting rest. She was the one mentioned in these pages who watched by poor Fisher's dying bed, and who won the especial love of all by the peculiarly holy calm that was ever round her. She was advanced in years, and had devoted her whole life to the service of God in deeds of charity.

She caught fever in her ward and was ill for one week. Great hopes were entertained of her recovery; but at last, she sank under her malady. One night in February the Sisters watched around the dying bed, a violent storm arose, which threatened to unroof the hut with every blast that swept over it, but she heard it not. Mingling with the tempest's roar went up the prayers for the dying, and as they bade the "*Christian soul depart in peace,*" she passed away, gentle in life—peaceful in death. The day following was Sunday; and in the evening they bore away the mortal remains of Sister Mary Elizabeth to lay them by the side of Sister Winefrede.

Before the funeral commenced, some of the *Soeurs de la Charité* from the Sardinian camp came with love and sympathy to their Sisters in Christ. Neither band knew the other's language, but united in the language of one common faith, they joined together in prayer. Soldiers of the 89th Regiment carried the coffin, followed by the Sisters, a Sister of Mercy and a Sister of Charity side by side. They passed through the double file of soldiers, all with heads uncovered. The coffin rested in the chapel, where seven priests chanted the burial service.

The chapel was crowded two hours before the service commenced. When the coffin was carried forth the concourse was immense. Medical officers and the Lady Superintendent of St. George's Hospital attended. It must have been pleasing to the Sisters under their affliction to witness the love and respect paid to the memory of their lost Sister by all.

A strange resting-place on the brow of that rugged hill is it for those two gentle Sisters. Around them lie the bodies of many who have fallen in deadly combat, and their too have fought a good fight, and have not been afraid to lay down their lives in Christ's service. They sought not the praise of men, and now they have found their reward—

For they beneath their Leader,
Who conquered in the fight,
For ever and for ever
Are clad in robes of white.

And now we will leave the Sisters of Mercy at Balaclava, trusting that God will keep them, and in His good time bring them home in safety.

The rejoicings for the blessings of peace will, we trust, ere long resound throughout the length and breadth of Europe, and thus will of necessity terminate the nursing in our Eastern hospitals. With an emergency it was suddenly organized, and will thus naturally find its end—but its effects will not so soon, we trust, pass away.

Attention has been drawn towards the class of women whose task it is to nurse the sick of England. These pages will in some degree show how unfitted they are for that responsible office. For though a military hospital was the worst imaginable position in which to place them, yet those who were unable to resist its temptations are certainly unfitted for their present occupation.

Regarding the ladies who went out various opinions have been entertained. Perhaps in this case their own view of their position may be the best, as they learnt their knowledge by experience, and most of them agreed that though in the great emergency that had nailed them forth their efforts had been blessed to the relief of much suffering, the system was based on no permanent footing. To raise the occupation of a nurse to a higher standard, to form a body who will both nurse in our home hospitals as well as be ready to attend the sick in the army and navy, other means are required.

There are two reasons which may be alleged against the permanent employment of ladies. For the arduous duties of an hospital (especially in a foreign country) long training is required ere the health can endure them. The neglect of this precaution will cause a waste of many valuable lives, while the amount of good for which they will be sacrificed will be but small.

Again, experience is necessary for the attainment of skill in nursing, and it is therefore necessary nurses should be changed as seldom as possible. But this is simply unavoidable when they are ladies possessing home ties and duties which they are only enabled temporarily to relinquish. Of course, there are exceptions to this as well as all other objections which may be raised against the plan, but I speak not of small or isolated efforts, I speak of a supply to the present great deficiency of nurses for the poor of England.

How small has been the number of women sent to the military hospitals of Scutari, Koulali, and Balaclava. 142 in all, (I do not speak of either Smyrna or Renkioi, with the numbers of whose nursing staff I am unacquainted), and of these only 55 were volunteers—27 ladies, 28 Sisters of Mercy, (there were thirty-three ladies in all, but six of these received payment); and of these only 17 ladies and 20 Sisters were on the spot at one time, while in the French and Sardinian services there have been hundreds of a *Soeurs de la Charité*.

But, I repeat, it is not for military hospitals alone that we want better nurses. War, it is hoped, has almost passed, and its trials and troubles too; but as long as this world continues, suffering will go on, and will prevail to its greatest extent among the poor; and shall England, who proudly boasts her superiority in science, government, and wealth above other nations, be behindhand in alleviating the bitter sufferings of her own children?

Many who will read these pages have perhaps never passed within hospital walls, many more, if they have done so, have paid their visit at appointed times when all looked its best. But others as well as myself have learnt our experience of hospital work from more authentic sources. We have *lived* in hospital wards, going there for the purpose of preparing ourselves—first, to undertake the nursing of the poor at home, and again when about to proceed to the East.

We placed ourselves under the hospital nurses, receiving our instruction from them, and, thus being possessed of no authority over them, were admitted behind the scenes of hospital life; and what we saw there— of disobedience to medical orders and cruelty to patients— would fill pages, and make those who read them shudder! shudder as we often have done when we saw some little innocent child, who from some terrible accident had been brought into the hospital, exposed to that atmosphere of evil. More evil was heard in one hour in a London hospital than would meet one's ears during months passed in a military one.

One word must be said for the nurses. Their work is no light one. The founder of the Sisters of Charity deemed that the attendance on all the loathsome diseases of mankind should exempt his daughters from practising any of those austerities which are enforced on religious communities. It is no easy task to bear with patience the endless fretfulness of hundreds of sick, to listen to long complaints with real sympathy, and speak soothing words when body and mind are alike worn.

To stand by the sufferer when about to undergo some fearful operation, to maintain a cheerful spirit when the familiar sounds are those of moans, of sufferings, or sharp cries of agony, while the very atmosphere is impregnated with disease. To be firm in carrying out the doctor's commands when they are a torture to the patients, and yet gentle and self-sacrificing in all that concerns themselves. While watchful care must be taken that familiarity with the sight and sound of suffering does not bring that hardening to it which is apt to creep over even a naturally tender nature, and which is one great cause of the cruelty and neglect practised by hospital nurses.

No, a good nurse must receive every new case of affliction as though it were her first. Yet all this and far more would be the portion of a hospital nurse. Can any believe that the love of gain or mere kindliness of heart can accomplish this? Generous impulses, enthusiasm, and benevolence, were called forth by stirring accounts of the suffering of our country's heroes, and bore many forth to struggle through a time which, like that of all passing distress, was one of great excitement; but the spirit that can go through long years of preparation—that can relinquish the fair things of this world to attend upon the grievously afflicted—must be the one of love springing from the sole desire to follow His steps, who came *"not to be ministered unto, but to minister."*

Memories of the Crimea

Contents

Preface	225
"Are There No Such Nurses in England?"	227
First Steps	231
Perils by Sea	235
"Not Wanted at Scutari"	237
In Hospital at Last	239
With the Sick and Wounded at Koulali	244
To Balaklava	247
Two Martyrs of Mercy	252
In and Out of Combat	259
Homeward Bound	266
After Many Days	269
Appendix	274

Preface

The narrative of the Crimean War has found its place in European history; and the story of its victories and defeats, of its glories and ghastly sufferings, have been eloquently told by both poets and historians. Yet, though the picture seemed complete in its interest and pathos, the following pages cast some new lights and darker shades on the incidents to which they refer, and impart to the whole an additional interest.

They tell of the hospitals—Scutari, Koulali, and Balaklava—filled to overflowing with the wounded and dying victims of the battlefield. And they also tell of many who were not the victims of shot or shell or sabre wound, but of the gaunt spectre of cholera or fever contracted by exposure in the trenches.

To minister to them was truly a noble field for the exercise of heroic Christian charity; and one that appealed to all that was generous and self-sacrificing in the nation. The present little volume shows how, from Ireland and England, heroic nuns went forth to minister to those dying soldiers, seeking and receiving no recompense save that which a God of charity has promised for what is done even for the least of His little ones. And the graves of Sisters Winifred and Elizabeth, still pointed out on the heights of Balaklava, speak with touching pathos of the character of their heroism.

Of the Irish Sisters who laboured in this merciful but perilous mission, one still survives at the Convent of Mercy, Gort, County Galway—the writer of this little book. Though weighted with the infirmities of age, she has yielded to the solicitations of friends, and given in these pages the graphic but simple history of her Crimean experiences. At a time when the ominous echoes of war resound once more through Europe from Eastern battlefields, the narrative must possess a special interest.

For the charity that will minister to the dying soldier, even at the risk of life, will ever command the admiration of all that is best in human nature. And it is gratifying to be able to add, that the distinction of the "Red Cross," recently conferred on the author of this work by our Gracious Queen, is a manifestation of our sovereign's appreciation of those services, without parallel in our history for over three hundred years.

J. Fahey, D.D., V.G.

Gort, County Galway,
Feast of Pentecost, 1897.

CHAPTER 1

"Are There No Such Nurses in England?"

One morning, as the Sisters were assembled for morning lecture in the Community Room of the Convent of Mercy, Carlow, the Reverend Mother read the following letter, received by the morning post from the Parent House of the Sisterhood, Baggot Street, Dublin:

My Dear Rev. Mother,
The Government has virtually applied for Sisters, and offered to pay their expenses; and as there is no time to be lost, I beg of you to send your candidates on Tuesday or Wednesday, to St. Catherine's, and if their service be not required, they can return. The eyes of the whole world will be on the poor nuns. I know you will select those that will give most glory to God. They will want a supply of clothing, etc. Five Sisters from Bermondsey have gone to the war as a private charity. Give all the aid you can, and believe me, my dear Rev. Mother, affectionately yours in Jesus Christ,

Sister M. Vincent Whitty,
Superioress.

Enclosed with this letter were the copies of two others. One, addressed by the same Superioress to the Vicar-General, the Very Rev. Dr. Yore:

Very Rev. Sir,
We have heard with great pain of the sufferings of our countrymen engaged as soldiers in the East in the service of the Queen. We know it must be difficult, if not impossible, to procure for them skilful nurses speaking their own language and sympathising with their habits and feelings, and that care and attention in a strange land which would be so well supplied at home. Attendance on the sick, as you are aware, is part of the work of our Institute, and sad experience amongst the poor has convinced us that, even with the advantages of medical aid,

many valuable lives are lost for want of careful nursing. It has occurred to us that as the French Sisters of Charity have been found so useful and acceptable to their countrymen in the hospitals of Constantinople, we, too, might render similar service to our countrymen, and help to mitigate their sufferings in the English hospitals.

We, therefore, Rev. Sir, through you, and with your permission, in the absence of the archbishop, beg leave to offer our services to the proper authorities to act as nurses in the care of the sick and wounded under the direction of the medical officers. Our services must necessarily be gratuitous. Only let us be transferred to the scene of our labours and be maintained there, and the survivors brought back to our own country.

Hoping to receive a favourable reply,
    I am, respectfully and sincerely,
        Yours in Jesus Christ,
            Sister Mary Vincent Whitty.

The other letter, from Dr. Yore to the Secretary of War, approving of the proposal, was as follows:

I have just received the enclosed letter from the Sisters of Mercy, making an offer of their services to attend our sick and wounded soldiers in the East. They have addressed the letter to me, in my character of Vicar-General and charged with the administration of the diocese in the absence of the archbishop. I need not say that their proposal has my hearty concurrence, and if the Government will accept of it, I shall be happy to give my best services in carrying it into effect. I do not anticipate that we shall be able at present to send more than from ten to twenty nuns, and it will be necessary that they be conveyed to the scene of their labours and maintained there, and that they be accompanied by a chaplain, who should continue during their stay and return with them, receiving the usual appointments of a chaplain.

When all the letters were read each Sister went to the choir, to visit the Blessed Sacrament, a custom which is usual after lecture or any notable event—and on their return any Sisters who wished to go were told to put their names into a little box left on the mantelpiece to receive them.

    I believe the whole community offered to go; but only two could be spared, and the two selected were Sister M. Aloysius and Sister M. Stanislaus, both young and healthy, and well accustomed to attend the sick poor of the town, which they did when cholera had raged a short time previously. Now the bishop's permission had to be got. He was very kind-hearted, and did not so easily give his sanction. He paced up and down the reception-room, saying:

> Out among soldiers, and perhaps on the field of battle too. I know they go out amongst the sick poor of the town, but this is quite a different thing.

However, after some time he gave his consent, with a fervent blessing and a promise of daily remembrance in the Holy Sacrifice—and endless injunctions to Rev. Mother to provide us with warm clothing and other comforts. But this solicitude was not needed, as no Community in the Order had a kinder Superior than St. Leo's had.

And now there is no time to be lost, we are to be ready to start when the telegram arrives from Baggot Street. We had to say goodbye to many a dear one outside the convent as well as within. Dr. Yore appointed Dr. Quinn, afterwards Bishop of Brisbane, to accompany two of the Baggot Street Sisters in search of volunteers for the Crimean Mission. Bishop Quinn often narrated this incident at the Antipodes. I give it in his own words:

> While sitting with a few agreeable friends I was informed that two ladies in a carriage outside wished to speak to me. I went immediately to ascertain who they were and what might be their business. I found they were two Sisters of Mercy, and after exchanging salutation, one said they would be obliged if I would get my hat and cloak and accompany them. I asked where to. She replied there was no time for explanation—they were already in danger of being late for the train, they would tell me on the way.
> It appeared that a number of Sisters of Mercy were wanted as nurses at the Crimea, and the Government applied to Dr. Manning to obtain them, and the two Sisters already mentioned were on their way to the South of Ireland to collect them. After travelling all night, we arrived at Kinsale very early in the morning. Having seen the Sisters to their Convent, I went to the church to perform my devotions. I soon fell into a sound sleep where I knelt, and so continued till aroused by the commotion of a number of persons around me. These good people

looked perplexed and alarmed at seeing a stranger, dressed as a priest, in such a helpless, inexplicable condition.

I felt bound to allay their concern by explaining how I came there. When the Rev. Mother M. Francis Bridgeman heard the business on which the Sisters had come, she sent to request that the bishop would be good enough to come down from Cork. He arrived within a few hours, and the whole Community, commencing with the Reverend Mother, begged on their knees to be allowed to join in the perilous expedition. All they saw in the dreadful accounts which had reached home from the Crimea was that it afforded a short cut to Heaven. The bishop allowed the Superioress and two Sisters to accompany us.

Were Dr. Quinn's relations with the Sisters unknown, it might appear that they treated him rather cavalierly in summoning him off so suddenly. In truth, he was a lifelong friend—from his ordination to his consecration he was chaplain or confessor to the Parent House; previous to the opening of the *Mater Misericordia*, he was appointed by Archbishop Cullen to accompany the three Sisters of Mercy who went to Amiens to study the hospital system in 1852, and made a tour of inspection of the principal hospitals in Europe, that the great hospital they projected might have the benefit of the most recent improvements, and that those destined to conduct it should have the fullest knowledge of hospital management.

The appeal from the East no Sister of Mercy could resist; and highly privileged did those deem themselves who were chosen for the enterprise. The hospitals were represented as filled with the dead and dying. The trenches were filled with the stark and stiffening corpses of many a frozen warrior; no food save the vilest could the brave men procure, very often no medicine, no attendance.

Reports of the condition of the wounded at Alma, September 20th, and at Inkerman, November 1st, 1854, horrified the humane, and wrung tears from the tender-hearted. Neither linen nor lint could be found to dress their gaping wounds; orderlies were their only nurses. Our allies did not suffer in this way. They summoned their Sisters on the first appearance of sickness, and the questions were constantly asked: "Are there no such nurses in England? Can the women do nothing for us in this fearful emergency?" But the women only waited to be asked. Lady M—— F——, the widowed daughter of an Irish nobleman, engaged three nurses, furnished money for their outfit and expenses, and offered to take them to the East herself should no one more competent be found. For the two thousand five hundred sick in the Scutari hospitals there were ten physicians, who certainly with the best intentions could not do much for these hapless patients.

But Baggot Street and Carlow were not the only Irish Convents in which this appeal of charity met with an immediate and practical response. We had some Sisters from Cork and Charleville. The response from Kinsale was equally prompt and generous; and thence came the Superioress, Mrs. Bridgeman, to whom the Sisters and the enterprise were greatly indebted.

CHAPTER 2

First Steps

The telegram came, and we were to start in the morning by the first train. Dr. Dunne, the President of Carlow College, said an early Mass, that we might have the happiness of receiving Holy Communion; and we began our journey accompanied by Rev. Mother, the Mother Assistant, and our respected friend, Dr. Dunne. We reached Baggot Street about eleven p.m., and surely, we got a loving greeting from the dear Sisters. Mother M.V.Whitty and Mother Xavier were as busy as they could be packing up.

They had heard so much about Turkey and its lazy inhabitants that they were afraid we could get nothing out there; so, they were determined to put in everything they could think of—soap, starch, smoothing irons, a medicine chest. As for warm clothing, there was no end of it. We might well call it the "Parent House"; and we, the band of Sisters of Mercy going out to the East, can never forgot their loving kindness.

Our future Rev. Mother, M. Francis Bridgeman, had already left for London with some of the Sisters; and we were to follow in the morning with other Sisters just arrived. And now the morning came, and we bade *adieu* to this truly happy Convent home. Reaching Kingstown about seven in the morning, we took our places in the steamer. There were great crowds waiting to see us off—"Sisters of Mercy *en route* for the seat of war"—and then, as the vessel moved off, a fervent "God speed you" arose in one loud cry.

Some of our party had to go to Blandford Square, others to the Convent of Mercy, Chelsea. The following letters, describing the journey and the reception in London, may perhaps bear insertion here:

My darling Rev. Mother,
We reached here last night about twelve o'clock, and were most affectionately greeted by Rev. Mother, who was expecting us. We had a very rough passage, and were very sick, but are now as well as ever, thank God. Our future Rev. Mother welcomed us this morning. Dear Sister M. Stanislaus is quite enthusiastic about her already. I must say I don't think we heard half good things enough about her: she seems to have both head and heart; and the Sisters here say she is a Saint as well. With such a Superioress we shall, with God's blessing, have a holy and successful mission.

We are getting such welcomes and pettings as we travel on that I fear we shall be spoiled if we ever return to dear St. Leo's. Our luggage is increasing so much that I think we shall have a good supply by the time we reach Turkey. I am very happy, and every day more and more-grateful to God for being one of the chosen few for the great work. Pray, dearest Mother, and, oh! do get the prayers of the dear Poor for your own
   Ever affectionate child in Jesus Christ,
              Sister M. Aloysius.
Thousands of loves to each of the dear Sisters.

And Sister M. Stanislaus wrote:

My dearest Rev. Mother,
I remained on deck while the vessel steamed out of Kingstown Harbour, to give, perhaps, a last look at my native hills, and feast my eyes once more on its beautiful bay. But my head began to reel, and I was obliged to adjourn to my cabin till the captain announced Holyhead. We soon took the train for London. Mr. Lucas, Editor of *The Tablet*, under whose care we had been placed by his relative, Mother V. Whitty, looked after our luggage, and was kind and attentive to us. When leaving us, we told him that we should offer a special prayer for him. He said he was sure we would on the score of universal charity, but he had no other claim. I am sure the Sisters in the old house at home will pray for him.

Will you, dear Rev. Mother, pray every day to the Blessed Virgin, that we may have health to discharge our duties to the poor, sick soldiers? If any of us got delicate at Scutari, it would be a great upset. Thank the dear Sisters a thousand times for all their kindness—the Rev. Mother and Sisters here are as kind and affectionate as if we were all their own. This morning we were introduced to our Eastern Mother—a fine, warm-hearted woman. I loved her the minute I saw her. Last night I prayed that I might like her, and that she might like me, and I think my prayer was granted.

Fond love to all, and believe me, my own dearest Rev. Mother, Your devoted child in Jesus Christ,

Sister M. Stanislaus.

This is the next note by the way:

Convent of Mercy, Chelsea, December1st, 1854.

My dearest Rev. Mother,

In the morning we leave London for our glorious mission. It will be carried on in a manner worthy of religion. Our dear Rev. Mother seems to have been specially selected for it. We travel in our veils, in the face of England—no disguise whatever. We are receiving gifts and blessings all day, and have scarcely time to ask who sends them.

Dr. Manning gave us a most beautiful exhortation this morning. How I wished you had heard him he is heart and soul in the mission, and said so many beautiful things about the amount of good to be effected that you would long to be of the happy band. You would think the Sister Missionaries all came from the one convent so united are they. Excuse this shabby note; my next will be from Paris.

Ever your devoted in Jesus Christ,

Sister M. Aloysius.

Notwithstanding the clear stipulations of Dr. Yore, there was some hesitation about our getting a chaplain—the authorities said if we got one, "the ladies should get one also." Rev. Mother said, "Why not give them one, if they desired it?" At last, Father Ronan, S.J., was named; and, perhaps, they could not have found one more fitted for the position. A fine, strong, young priest, cheerful and good; this appointment gave general satisfaction. Next, Rev. Mother was installed in her office by the London Vicar-General, Dr. Whitty (Cardinal Wiseman having left for Rome). Dr. Manning came to say goodbye and give us a last blessing. Lady Herbert came too— she was extremely nice. They told us that she was on the high road to Catholicity. (Wife of the Secretary of State for War. She became a Catholic shortly afterwards.)

On the morning of the 2nd of December, 1854, we left this dear, happy Convent, and its cherished inmates, who gave such a welcome to their Sisters from the Emerald Isle, and reached London Bridge Station long before dawn, where we formed part of as curious a group as ever London Bridge had witnessed. The ladies and paid nurses wore the same costume, and a very ugly one it was. It seemed to be contract work, and all the same size, so that the ladies who were tall had short dresses, and the ladies who were small had long dresses. They consisted of grey tweed wrappers, worsted jackets, white caps, and short woollen cloaks, and, to conclude, a frightful scarf of brown holland, embroidered in red with the words, "Scutari Hospital." That ladies could be found to walk into such a costume was certainly a triumph of grace over nature.

We started from Portsmouth, and we reached Boulogne about one o'clock p.m. The Sisters of the Ursuline Convent had some of the boarders to meet us with an invitation to lunch, but there was not time for that. The poor fisherwomen greeted us most warmly on our way to the hotel for lunch. The host and hostess got quite beside themselves at having fifteen veiled nuns in their house. It appears that all the French veiled nuns are cloistered. They would not take money for our refreshments.

As we travelled on, sad news reached us from the seat of war—thousands, wounded and dying, in the hospitals. Paris, we reached very late. Next day, Sunday, we heard Mass, and got Holy Communion at the Church of *Notre Dame des Victoires*. At two o'clock we went to Vespers, and we remained till four.

Miss Stanley, who had charge of the party, was untiring in her attention to us. (The sister of Dean Stanley.) She too became a devout member of the Catholic Church. Next morning, after an early Mass, we took the train for Lyons, travelling all day. The whole country looked like a pleasure-ground, laid out by the hand of a more than terrestrial gardener. Green hills, rising above each other, gave a delightful effect to the richly cultivated valleys. Here lay acres devoted to the vine, there rose the lofty cypress, the mulberry, and the cedar.

We passed Dijon, saw the church in which St. Francis de Sales preached and was first seen by St. Jane Frances de Chantal. We drove through a shallow part of the Seine, Loire, and Rhone, and reached Lyons about ten at night. We drove to the hotel, where an immense crowd awaited to see us. We were a great curiosity; such a large party, and in such different costumes, all going to the seat of war.

Next morning, we had the unspeakable happiness of getting Mass and Holy Communion, owing to the kindness of Miss Stanley, who seems to know the hours and customs as we travel on. She has been nearly all over the world, which is a great advantage to us. Immediately after breakfast we started by boat for Valence. Our first accident occurred here. The boat struck on a sand-bank, and it took several hours to raise her. We did not proceed direct to Marseilles, as we intended. It was late when we arrived at Avignon—we were shown to the hotel which is supposed to be the palace occupied by the Popes during their stay in the city.

Here Miss Stanley was quite at home. Never can we forget the hostess's attention. Indeed, all through France we had met with the greatest kindness. We got two Masses next morning. In Marseilles, where we ended our railway travelling, we rose early next morning and spent a long time in the church.

Chapter 3

Perils by Sea

About three o'clock in the afternoon we took our places in an old French vessel called the *Egyptus*. The gentlemen of the party were not quite satisfied with it, but it was the only one available. It was crammed with cavalry bound for the seat of war. The day was wild and stormy, and the night was one to be long remembered. One of the sailors said the devil raised the storm, but that "Mary would calm it." It took some hours to get everything right: at last, the vessel moved. I do not think there was ever such a medley in any ship as in the old *Egyptus* that memorable evening.

We kept as much as possible on deck. We passed the Straits of Bonifacio and the Straits of Messina—land visible on both sides. The Italian mountains, enclosing all so Catholic, were particularly attractive, but were surpassed in beauty by Sicily. We anchored at Messina for some time, with the permission of the governor. The scene, viewed from the ship, was enchanting. The ladies brought us some boughs from the convent bearing their golden oranges. Boats passed and repassed from our ship to the shore; the Sicilians rowing over oranges and figs, which were purchased and liberally distributed to all on board. A poor woman continued cruising around the vessel all day, singing a hymn to the Madonna for charity, which was freely bestowed on her.

We set sail again and left behind us the comfort and security of *terra firma*. The night was very fine; but next day, about eleven o'clock, a most terrific storm arose, accompanied by rain, thunder, and lightning—and then the night—oh, such a frightful night, and how dark! The top was blown off the cabin; the engineer's hut washed off deck. The vessel, now so long on one side, would suddenly turn over with such a fearful crash that we expected every moment would be our last; but dear Rev. Mother, whose courage never failed, told us, over and over again, that there was no fear; that our Heavenly Father never took us from our convent homes to leave us in the bottom of the Mediterranean; that He had more work for us to do—in a word, that we were not going to get the crown so easily. The captain put in next day to Navarino, for shelter and repairs.

The ninth day of our voyage we anchored on the shore of old Athens. The coast is some distance from the old town. The day being beautifully fine, with the aid of a glass we could see the Areopagus and other places of note. Many Athenians came on board, in costume very like that of the Highlanders. An Athenian priest came to visit us, and on his return sent two Sisters of Charity to see us, bringing a present of oranges and flowers.

One of the Sisters was Irish—a great and unexpected pleasure. She was charmed to meet nuns from the Emerald Isle. The other was French, and got a welcome from the French soldiers, who gathered round to show their respect for the daughter of St. Vincent de Paul. The Sisters had no convent at Athens, but came from Smyrna to attend cholera patients.

We set sail again, and the captain said we should have fine weather for the rest of the voyage. At last, we neared our destination. The hills of Armenia became visible. We were overjoyed to see any portion of a place so dear and memorable to us. Passing the plains of old Troy and many other places of note, we entered the Dardanelles, past fortifications, and any number of gipsy tents—they pitch their tents in the old vessels along the coast.

We cast anchor at a little town called Gallipoli, where the English troops first landed: there was a hospital for the English. Two Sisters of Charity embarked on their way to Galata, a suburb of Constantinople, where their Convent was, the Mother House of their Order in the East. And then, thank God, we arrived quite safely on shore at the Turkish capital.

Chapter 4

"Not Wanted at Scutari"

The delight of seeing the magnificent city of Constantinople, after long and irksome confinement in a cabin, can scarcely be conceived. Those marble palaces and domes rising out of the placid waters of the Bosphorus into the lovely blue of an Eastern sky—turn your eyes where you will, and you see one thing more lovely than another. From all we had heard and read, the Turks alone seem out of place in this Garden of Eden.

But, as we were expecting every hour to embark, messages had been sent to Scutari; but no reply had come. The vessel had to be cleared of passengers and luggage at no distant hour, when, at last, strange news for the nuns arrived:

"Not wanted at Scutari."

The War Office had made a mistake in sending out the party—no room for them! We were astonished, and no wonder: in a strange country, and among very strange people. What were we to do? Dear Rev. Mother, who was always calm in the midst of difficulties, wrote to the Sisters of Charity at Galata, asking hospitality for a short time, till she could see her way as to the future. Miss Stanley applied to the British Embassy for her party. In a wonderfully short time, we saw two of the French Sisters coming over to our ship in a boat. And were they not welcome?

They brought a loving greeting from their Superior. At once they saw after our luggage; and a large boat from one of the war vessels came to bring us ashore. We had to pass through Constantinople, and we knew that *"All is not gold that glitters."* We had not expected anything quite so bad as what met our view in the narrow filthy streets. And now, what shall I say of the dear, kind Rev. Mother of the French Sisters at Galata, who waited in the hall to welcome her fifteen guests? She did so with as much affection as if we were all her own children. We were one in faith, and in that far off country we were able to join in the prayers and devotions as if we were in the dear little chapel of St. Leo's, Carlow.

They first brought us to the choir, which was to us a third Heaven. There, before our Divine Lord, many a fervent prayer was said. He knew all our hearts, and how earnestly we desired to be at the work which we came to do. We were then shown into a large schoolroom, which had just been emptied of children to accommodate us. We were naturally pained at putting the Community to so much inconvenience; but in their own kind and cheerful way they did their best to make us feel quite at home.

Many of our Sisters spoke French fluently, so that we had no difficulty in that way. The Sisters had a private chapel, but there was also a large church attached to the Convent, which belongs to the Lazarists or Vincentian Fathers—some French, others Armenians. In Galata, the poorest division of Constantinople, the French and Catholic Armenians principally resided.

It was Christmas Eve at the Convent of Galata. The little chapel was adorned with flowers and candles. We had midnight Mass, a great pleasure to us; and then all the fuss and preparation reminded us of our own dear Convent. Before Mass we had a most interesting ceremony—the reception into the Church of an Eastern princess, granddaughter to the Bey of Algiers. On Christmas morning we had six Masses and Benediction—our first Christmas Day in the East.

I must now say something of the duties of these Sisters of Charity. They had large schools, containing sixty boarders—including Russians and twelve African slaves from the Soudan. They visited the sick poor in their homes, and brought them all the comfort they could. Their work in the hospitals was well known.

In a word, there was nothing too difficult for those self-sacrificing Sisters, where Gods glory was concerned; and then, when the active duties of the day were over, their spirit of prayer was wonderful. They combined the active and contemplative life perfectly. We were all deeply impressed by the fervour of these dear daughters of St. Vincent de Paul.

I must say a few words, too, about the French Naval Hospital, where we heard Mass while waiting for our chaplain, who did not arrive for nearly a month after us. The wards of this beautiful hospital were divided by glass partitions, and when the door of the pretty little chapel was opened every patient had a view of the altar, and could assist at Mass without the slightest inconvenience; it was most consoling to see how carefully the spiritual and temporal wants of the patients were attended to.

On Sunday four of the young cadets served at Mass, and presented arms at the Elevation. They were very polite and kind to us. Indeed, the comfort and care told on the patients—they looked calm and happy.

CHAPTER 5

In Hospital at Last

Christmas over, we hourly expected some news from headquarters. We longed to be at the work, and every day we heard that the poor soldiers were dying by hundreds, and we idle and close at hand. Rev. Mother was in correspondence with the authorities; and at last, a despatch came to say that five Sisters were to proceed to Scutari, to the General Hospital; while arrangements were made for the other ten Sisters to proceed to a house on the Bosphorus, to await further orders.

At once the five Sisters started for Scutari: Rev. Mother, Sister M. Agnes, Sister M. Elizabeth, Sister M. Winifred, and myself. When we reached Scutari, we were shown to our quarters, consisting of one little room, not in a very agreeable locality. However, we were quite satisfied none better could be found, and for this little nook we were very thankful.

Of course, we expected to be sent to the wards at once. Sister M. Agnes and the writer were sent to a store, to sort clothes that had been eaten by the rats; Rev. Mother and Sister M. Elizabeth either to the kitchen or to another store. In a dark, damp, gloomy shed we set to work and did the best we could; but, indeed, the destruction accomplished by the rats was something wonderful.

On the woollen goods they had feasted sumptuously. They were running about us in all directions; we begged of the sergeant to leave the door open that we might make our escape if they attacked us. Our home rats would run if you "hushed" them; but you might "hush" away, and the Scutari rats would not take the least notice.

During my stay in the stores, I saw numberless funerals pass by the window. Cholera was raging, and how I did wish to be in the wards amongst the poor dying soldiers! Before I leave the stores, I must mention that Sister M. Agnes and myself thought the English nobility must have emptied their wardrobes and linen stores to send out bandages for the wounded—the most beautiful underclothing, the finest cambric sheets, with merely a scissors run here and there through them to ensure their being used for no other purpose.

And such large bales, too; some from the Queen's Palace, with the Royal monogram beautifully worked. Whoever sent out these immense bales thought nothing too good for the poor soldiers. And they were right—nothing was too good for them. And now goodbye stores and goodbye rats; for I was to be in the cholera wards in the morning.

Where shall I begin, or how can I ever describe my first day in the hospital at Scutari? Vessels were arriving, and the orderlies carrying the poor fellows, who, with their wounds and frost-bites, had been tossing about on the Black Sea for two or three days, and sometimes more. Where were they to go? Not an available bed. They were laid on the floor one after another, till the beds were emptied of those dying of cholera and every other disease. Many died immediately after being brought in—their moans would pierce the heart—the taking of them in and out of the vessels must have increased their pain.

The look of agony in those poor dying faces will never leave my heart. They may well be called "The Martyrs of the Crimea." We went round with hot wine, and relieved them in every way as far as it was possible. We went to the Catholic soldiers, took the names of those in immediate danger, that the chaplain might go to them at once. He was there; but it hastened matters for him to get the list of worst cases. The beds were by degrees getting empty. If stretchers were bringing in some from the vessels, others were going out with the dead. We were able to get the men on the floor to bed; then, of course, we could see after them better.

The cholera was of the very worst type—the attacked man lasted only four or five hours. Oh! those dreadful cramps; you might as well try to bend a piece of iron as to move the joints. The medical staff did their best, and daily, hourly risked their own lives, with little or no success. At last, every one seemed to be getting paralysed, and the orderlies indifferent as to life or death.

The usual remedies ordered by the doctors were stuping and poultices of mustard. They were very anxious to try chloroform, but they did not trust anyone with it except the Sisters. Rev. Mother was a splendid nurse, and had the most perfect way of doing everything. For instance, the stuping seems such a small thing, but if not properly done it did more harm than good. I will give her way. You have a large tub of boiling water, blankets torn in squares, and a piece of canvas with a running at each end to hold a stick.

The blankets were put into the boiling water, lifted out with a tongs and put into the canvas, when an orderly at each end wrung the flannel out so dry that not a drop of water remained, before a preparation of chloroform was sprinkled on it, and it was applied to the stomach. Then followed a spoonful of brandy, and immediately after a small piece of ice, to try to settle the stomach, and finally rubbing with mustard, and even with turpentine. Rarely, very rarely, did any remedy succeed; and, as a rule, it was not the weak or delicate who were attacked, but the strong and healthy.

One day a fine young fellow, the picture of health and strength, was carried in on a stretcher to my ward. I said to the orderlies, "I hope we shall be able to bring *him* through."

I set to work with the usual remedies; but the doctor shook his head, and said: "I am afraid it's all no use, Sister."

When the orderlies, poor fellows, were tired, I set to work myself, and kept it on till nearly the end—but you might as well rub iron; no heat, no movement from his joints. He lived about the usual time—four or five hours.

A hurried line to my convent home, St. Leo's, Carlow, ran as follows:

> Scutari Hospital,
> January, 1855.
>
> My dearest Rev. Mother,
>
> You are, no doubt, very anxious for some news of your two dear ones now so far away. I am here, at the place so often talked of. And what am I doing? If you could only get one look at this dreadful place it would never leave your mind or heart; but you would be consoled to see the Sisters in the midst of so much suffering. The hospital consists of long corridors, as far as your eye can reach, with beds at each side; and, as I write, poor fellows, both wounded and frost-bitten, lie on the floor. We are in the wards late and early. When we go to our apartment, to get a couple of hours rest, we groan in anguish at the thought of all we have undone.
>
> Pray, pray much for us, my own dear Mother. In great haste,
>
> Your ever fond,
>
> M. Aloysius.
>
> I really grudge the few minutes I have taken to write this—don't expect letters.

Week in, week out, the cholera went on. The same remedies were continued, though almost always to fail. However, while there was life there was hope, and we kept on the warm applications to the last. When it came near the end, the patients got into a sort of collapse, out of which they did not rally.

We begged the orderlies, waiting to take them to the dead-house, to wait a little lest they might not be dead; and with great difficulty we prevailed on them to make the least delay. As a rule, the orderlies drank freely, "to drown their grief," they said. I must say their position was a very hard one—their work always increasing—and such work; death around them on every side; their own lives in continual danger—it was almost for them a continuation of the field of battle.

The poor wounded men brought in out of the vessels were in a dreadful state of dirt; and so weak that whatever cleaning they get had to be done cautiously. Oh, the state of those fine fellows, so worn out with fatigue, so full of vermin! Most or all of them required spoon-feeding. We had wine, sago, arrowroot. Indeed, I think there was everything in the stores; but it was so hard to get them. We went every morning with the orderlies to get the wine, brandy, and other things ordered by the doctors: we gave them out according to their directions.

The medical officers were kind enough to say they had no one to depend on but the nuns. Sometimes, if allowed, the man might drink in one draught the brandy ordered for the day, which, of course, would do him great harm. An orderly officer took the rounds of the wards every night, to see that all was right. He was expected by the orderlies, and the moment he raised the latch one cried out: "All right, your honour."

Many a time I said "All wrong." The poor officer, of course, went his way; and one could scarcely blame him for not entering those wards, so filled with pestilence, the air so dreadful that to breathe it might cost him his life. And then what could he do even if he did come? I remember one day an officer's orderly being brought in—a dreadful case of cholera; and so devoted was his master that he came in every half-hour to see him, and stood over him in the bed as if it was only a cold he had; the poor fellow died after a few hours' illness. I hope his devoted master escaped. I never heard.

It was said that the graves were not made deep enough, and that the very air was putrid. There were no coffins, canvas and blankets had to suffice.

I must say something of my poor frostbitten patients. The men who came from the "Front," as they called it, had only thin linen suits—no other clothing to keep out the Crimean frost of 1854-1855. When they were carried in on the stretchers, which conveyed so many to their last resting-place, their clothes had to be cut off. In most cases the flesh and clothes were frozen together; and, as for the feet, the boots had to be cut off bit by bit—the flesh coming off with them—many pieces of the flesh I have seen remain in the boot. Poultices were applied with some oil brushed over them. In the morning, when these were removed—can I ever forget it?—the sinews and bones were seen to be laid bare.

We had surgical instruments; but in almost every case the doctors or staff-surgeons were at hand, and removed the diseased flesh as tenderly as they could. As for the toes, you could not recognise them as such. Far, far worse and more painful were these than the gun or sword wounds; and what must it have been where they had both? And then the poor frost-bitten fellows were so prostrate—no matter what care most of them got, they could not survive. One poor frost-bitten soldier told us that when, lying ill at Balaklava one night, he tried to stir his feet, he found them frozen to those of another soldier whose feet were lying against his.

A letter written by a Sister at the time will best continue the narrative at this point:

> We have just received some hundreds of poor creatures, worn out with sufferings beyond any you could imagine, in the Crimea, where the cold is so intense that a soldier described to me the Russians and the Allies in a sudden skirmish, and neither party able to draw a trigger! So, fancy what the poor soldiers must endure in the "trenches."

It is a comfort to think that these brave men had some care, all that we could procure for them. For at this time the food was very bad—goats' flesh, and something they called mutton, but black, blue, and green. Yet who could complain of anything after the sufferings I have faintly described—borne, too, with such patience: not a murmur!

The Catholic soldiers had every consolation of their religion; the chaplains, untiring, were late and early in the wards. Of course, we were free to say prayers for them, and, whenever we could, a word of instruction or consolation. One day, after a batch had arrived from the Crimea, and I had gone my rounds through them, one of my orderlies told me that a man wanted to speak one word to me.

When I had a moment, I went to him. "Tell me at once what you want; I have worse cases to see after"—he did not happen to be very bad.

"All I want to know, Ma'am, is, are you one of our own Sisters of Mercy from Ireland?"

"Yes," I said, "your very own."

"God be praised for that!"

Another poor fellow said to me one day, "Do they give you anything good out here?"

"Oh yes," I said, "why do you ask me?"

"Because, Ma'am, you gave me a piece of chicken for my dinner, and I kept some of it for you"—he pulled it out from under his head and offered it to me.

I declined the favour with thanks—I never could say enough of those kind-hearted soldiers and their consideration for us in the midst of their own sufferings.

CHAPTER 6

With the Sick and Wounded at Koulali

I shall now return to the Sisters from whom we parted at Galata. The day five of us left for Scutari the other ten took up their abode at Therapia, on the Asiatic side of the Bosphorus, about eight miles from Constantinople. The house belonged to the British Embassy. The ambassador's house was very near where Miss Stanley and her party were staying. The Sisters, all so anxious to be at work, were storming Heaven with prayers, and at last news arrived that a new hospital must be opened—there were such numbers coming from the Crimea and nowhere to put them.

There was a Turkish barracks in a lovely place on the banks of the Bosphorus, called Koulali, in which there were Russian prisoners. They were removed, poor fellows, I don't know where—and the barrack was given for a hospital. Attached to all Turkish barracks there is a hospital, and this also was given.

The first batch of sick and wounded that arrived numbered four hundred and ninety; and, perhaps, such desolate, worn-out looking patients never before entered any hospital. Dear Miss Stanley, who had been all along such a kind friend to the Sisters, entered heart and soul into the work. Miss Hutton, who was named as the Superintendent, was only too glad to hand it over to the Sisters, of whom five were apportioned to each hospital, giving a secular lady, nurses, and a Sister in each ward.

In the beginning there was great rubbing and scrubbing to make the wards anything like those of an English hospital; and so successfully that the ladies, the doctors, and nurses were all delighted; while, as for the orderlies, they used to look round in great delight and exclaim. "There is nothing like it anywhere."

Father Ronan, S. J., the chaplain, quickly gained the love of all classes: he was so kind with the soldiers, and perhaps there are no people in the world more grateful than they. There was any amount of real, genuine goodness under those red coats, or, as we had them out there, those poor linen suits. The work of the hospital went on beautifully. The doctors themselves called it the "Model hospital of the East."

Some thousands passed through the hospital during the Sisters' time there. The liberality of the soldiers adorned the chapel, where there was daily Mass. Convalescent patients thronged to the daily Mass; men off duty came when it was possible; and the Sisters had the satisfaction of knowing that no Catholic ever left Koulali without receiving the Sacraments, nor did a single Catholic die without the Church's consolations.

There was the greatest harmony between the Sisters and the ladies; but Miss Stanley, Miss Taylor, and Miss Hutton had the first place in their hearts. Miss Stanley and Miss Taylor were High Church Anglicans coming out; but before Miss Stanley returned to England she had been received into the Church by Father Ronan, thus yielding to her convictions against her old inclinations.

From all that I have seen and heard of the English, I believe, once they are convinced, they will step over every difficulty to do what they believe to be right. Miss Taylor was also received into the Church by the same priest, who received others also; while many of the poor soldiers who had fallen away from the Faith were by him restored to the grace and friendship of God. Miss Hutton was Low Church; but Rev. Mother, who had continual intercourse with her, often told us that she had never had dealings with a more honourable and upright mind. It was now Easter, and Miss Stanley must soon say goodbye to "her dear fifteen," as she called us—she came out only in charge of the party, and had delayed her return longer than she intended.

During the stay of the Sisters at this favoured spot they had a visit from the Purveyor-in-Chief, Mr. Scott Robinson. He was a Scotsman, and, before he paid us a visit, he had taken a survey of the hospitals. The ladies, nearly all, were ill; the nurses sick, too, and gone home; and it appeared, as he stated, that it was the Sisters who were doing the work of the hospital. He called on Rev. Mother one day, and requested to see our quarters. She at once showed him everything, and he expressed surprise that we were so badly lodged.

At once he went through the hospital, even to the doctors' quarters, and made us out much better accommodation. He placed entirely at our discretion all the stores, food, and clothing, and told Rev. Mother to act as if the hospital were her own. He said that we need not trouble ourselves any more about reports to the War Office, and that he would answer for us.

The weather was fearfully hot at this time, and insects of all kinds abounded—fleas, flies, bugs, ants, mosquitoes. As for rats, dogs, and donkeys, they were innumerable, and you may imagine how hard it was to get a sleep. Among other disquietudes, there was a gunpowder explosion, and the two hospitals were near being blown up.

Moreover, we had several shocks of earthquakes. I was in one of the wards, and suddenly felt the ground move under me, as if I stood on the waves of the sea. After this was a sudden trembling, and the windows began to shake with a strange noise; pictures, a clock, and other things, fell in the ward. The poor patients were terrified. There was an open square in the centre of the building, and all made a rush to get there; you may imagine what a scene it was—some hobbling, some tottering, and in their various degrees of undress. The shock lasted three minutes. We had another during the night—oh! such a strange and thrilling sensation, something like an electric shock.

When Miss Stanley reached England Her Majesty the Queen (anxious, of course, to hear all about her soldiers) sent for her; and when the interview was nearly over Her Majesty asked her what she thought the poor soldiers would like—she was anxious to send them a present.

****

Miss Stanley afterwards organised in London a Home, a lodging-house for women, a laundry at Westminster, a penny savings' bank, a society to distribute flowers to the poor and hospitals— and a contracting agency, at her own risk, for Government clothing, whereby work was supplied to soldiers' widows and other poor women. She rendered besides valuable service during the Cotton Famine; also, to the Society for Aid to the Sick and Wounded. She had a great heart for the poor soldiers: she thought nothing was too good for them; and she was right.

****

Miss Stanley said: "Oh, I do know what they would like—plenty of flannel shirts, mufflers, butter, and treacle." Her Majesty said they must have all these things; and they did come out in abundance: Koulali got its share of the gifts. But the very name of butter or treacle was enough for the doctors: they said they would not allow it into the wards, because it would be going about in bits of paper and daubing everything. So, Rev. Mother at once interposed, and said if the doctors allowed it, she would have it distributed in a way that could give no trouble. They apologised, and said they should have known that, and at once left everything to her.

Each Sister got her portion of butter and treacle (which were given only to the convalescent patients), and when the bell rang every evening for tea she stood at the table in the centre of the ward and each soldier walked over and got his bread buttered and some treacle if he wished spread on like jam. We told them it was a gift from the queen; and if Her Majesty could only have seen how gratified they were it would have given her pleasure. One evening Lady Stratford, and some distinguished guests who were staying at the Embassy, came, and were much pleased to see how happy and comfortable the men were, and how much they enjoyed Her Majesty's gifts.

Chapter 7

To Balaklava

Now I come back to Scutari, which was the principal scene of my labours. The cholera continued during the summer months, with less terrible results; but typhus fever broke out in its worst form. Every bed was occupied: I was assisted by a lady, two nurses, and orderlies. Everyone knows the nursing that is required in cases of fever. The constitutions of the men were so undermined that they were not able to endure any sickness. Each day we had a number of deaths, and each day others took the dead men's places—themselves to die.

Some kind friends sent out a quantity of aromatic vinegar, of which there was some in the stores also; this was the greatest refreshment the poor patients got. When a little of it was put into water, and they were sponged with it over and over, they used to hold out their poor hands for more. My lady companion in the ward (Miss Smythe) caught the fever and lived only one week. It was hard on these ladies, many of whom, I suppose, had left luxurious homes, and were totally unaccustomed to that kind of work, some of them never having seen a dead man before.

They often regretted that they had no experience, and they leaned on us in every difficulty. Sisters of Mercy have a novitiate of four and a-half years, during which they are exercised in various works of mercy; so, to them it was no new thing to face disease and death. To live for the Poor had been for many years the resolve of each heart. Trained as we had been, the health and strength of the Sisters withstood the shock under which the health of the ladies sank. No wonder that Miss Nightingale should lean on Mother Mary Clare, of Bermondsey, and her four Sisters, who were with her at the Barrack Hospital. (See Appendix for fuller notes about the work of the contingent of nuns and nurses from the Bermondsey Convent.)

Even the health of our dear and valued friend, Father Ronan, began to fail, and he was ordered home by the doctors, to the regret of poor patients as well as our own, and that of the officers with whom he messed. But as the patients at Koulali were by that time nearly all convalescent, we felt that we might soon be going ourselves. We had some kind friends among the Protestant clergy; others of them seemed to be watching our every movement. We could not help feeling that they regarded us with great suspicion, and we often got letters from the War Office which we felt were owing to their reports.

The letters used to amuse us very much; they accused us of interfering with the religion of the Protestant soldiers, and informed us that we were only nurses—that St. Paul said women were not to preach or to teach! Dear Rev. Mother would not feel put out by reports of that kind—she knew well that the War Office was misinformed, and that the truth would triumph. It is not our way to force the conscience of anyone. Even if we had never promised the War Office not to interfere with them, the Protestant soldiers had been quite safe.

The Holy Spirit alone can enlighten the soul. Nor did the millions of tracts sent out from England, and freely distributed amongst the Catholic soldiers, gain one "convert." One of the Protestant patients said one day: "I care not for creed or difference of opinion—to me you are all angels of mercy, and on behalf of my comrades and myself I express my gratitude."

One day the sergeant-major of a Highland regiment was carried in on a stretcher. He had been drinking. The doctor examined him, and did not order him any stimulants. When the time came that the stimulants were being given out in the ward, he was inconsolable to find there was none for him. He was just getting out of delirium, and he told me that if he did not get a little, he would not be alive next day. He said the doctor was young, and did not understand his complaint.

I thought myself that it was absolutely necessary for him; so, I went to the doctor and asked him to allow me to give him a little. He said:

"Very well, Sister, let it be only a little."

We became great friends. He was sent home as an invalid; and when he was carried from the ward, he raised himself up on the stretcher and cried out: "I thank you, my blessed lady; but for you I should be in my grave. May my blessing and the blessing of God be with you!"

There was no use in my telling him that the title he addressed to me was one given only to the Queen of Heaven. In a word, we found the Protestant soldiers only too grateful and respectful.

One of the friendly Protestant clergymen, most of them very nice and polite, responded to our wish to be on happy terms with them, and asked Rev. Mother where she got her clothes so beautifully made up. She told him one of our lay-Sisters did them. "Well," he said, "I am in a wretched state about my collars." She at once offered to get them done for him. Others followed suit: with much pleasure she got them all done. We never heard that any of the Protestant ladies who worked with us in the wards made an unkind remark of us, save one Miss A.—who made a charge against us that we were "proselytising." So, Rev. Mother, with her usual decision, at once determined to see the lady and hear all about it. She did so, and the following is the conversation that was held:

Rev. Mother: "I am informed, Miss A., that you assert that, to your own knowledge, the Sisters are interfering with the religion of the Protestants?"

Miss A.: "Yes, I do, to my own knowledge."

Rev. Mother: "Well, pray tell me in what instance and in what ward did it happen?"

Miss A.: "In Dr. Psalter's."

Rev. Mother: "And with what Sister?"

Miss A.: "I am sure I don't know."

Rev. Mother: "What was the man's name?"

Miss A.: "I don't know—I forget."

Rev. Mother: "What was the nature of the instruction?"

Miss A.: "I did not ask. The man said to me one day that he was complaining of not seeing the minister, that only for the Popish Nuns he would know nothing about his religion; that they sent their priest into the ward three times a day. That was all he said."

Rev. Mother: "And how could that lead you to suppose that the Sisters had been speaking to him on religion?"

Miss A.: "I don't know; but I thought they had done so."

The Superintendent, Miss Hutton, was present, and said she could not help feeling disgusted with the accusation. Yet we knew very well that the War Office would never send us out such preambles and preachments if they were not being misinformed.

At last, the Koulali hospitals were to be given up to the allied Sardinian troops—the patients being all convalescent, and the hospitals at the "Front" sufficient to accommodate the present sick and wounded. Meanwhile, Rev. Mother had been in correspondence with Sir John Hall, the principal medical officer in the East, about our going to Balaklava, to take charge of a hospital of which, he said, Miss Nightingale had given up the charge. Both he and the Purveyor-in-Chief were most anxious that we should make no delay; and on the 7th of October, 1855, we left both Scutari and Koulali, on board the *Ottawa*, bound for Balaklava. Sir J. Hall made the arrangements for our voyage.

We did not leave Scutari or Koulali without regret. In the latter, particularly, we had kind friends amongst the ladies and doctors. And what shall I say about the poor soldiers who had been under our care for so many months, and our devoted orderlies? Indeed, I think I may say with truth that we left amidst the prayers and blessings of all and the tears of many. Father Woollett, S.J., came to fetch us. The morning of our departure all our little commodities were packed up; and the doctors came to our quarters laden with good things for our breakfast—toasted bacon, eggs, and jam. At last, the goodbye was said to this dear spot, and we proceeded to the vessel.

We passed the Embassy, and Lady Stratford and many others greeted us as we sailed off, accompanied by Father Woollett. On the morning of the 10th of October, we were in view of the heights of Balaklava, and just at the mouth of the harbour. Signals were hoisted to see if we might enter. The entrance is between immense rocks, and the passage so very narrow that only one vessel can enter at a time. The harbour itself forms a basin.

Hours passed, and the signal had not been responded to. Besides, there were other vessels before us, waiting for admittance. Anchor could not be cast on account of the rocks, and out in the Black Sea we were likely to spend the night. We could hear the sound of the cannon and shell doing their work of destruction. In truth, we were at that moment where we would never be but "*For Heaven, Lord, and Thee.*"

At last, about six in the evening, an express came to say that a tug was lying hard by to convey us ashore. It lay some distance from the ship, and could only be reached by our ship boat. The waves were mountains high when the boat came alongside. Rev. Mother was on deck, and at once she stepped In, accompanied by Sister M. Joseph, Father Woollett, and a Protestant clergyman from Koulali.

Miss Nightingale, who had come up from Scutari, was on board; and as soon as the tug had left its first burthen ashore it returned to take her and the rest of the Sisters over. The captain, however, thought it safer to put to sea than to venture over; so, we did not find ourselves landed in the harbour of Balaklava till eight next evening. Father Woollett, S.J., was waiting to bring us to our quarters. The way to our hut was up a steep hill. The hut was made of wood, not too closely put together; there was a door, and above the door a window, and another window at the opposite end. A new hut was to be erected for us; but these arrangements were very slowly carried out.

When we reached the hut, Rev. Mother welcomed us as if it was to a palace. She had a cloth spread on the floor, and two orderlies were looking after our dinner. I am sure we never enjoyed anything so much as this our first dinner in the Crimea—our dear Mother was ever so well, and as happy and cheerful as any of us. We had no ladies or nurses in Balaklava: all the nursing, day and night, was to be done by the Sisters. The poor orderlies got us our dinner, something, they said, like mutton; but the sheep had come from Malta, and were nearly dead from hunger and hardship before they reached the Crimea.

When Sir John Hall heard of our arrival, he came and welcomed us, and gave us the charge of the General Hospital, in which we had the use of one small room. Fifteen or sixteen huts had patients in each of them. The huts were very straggling; and at this time the mud was something dreadful. Who has not heard of the mud of Balaklava? It increased the labour very much.

When we began our work, we discovered that the soldiers had had some little care bestowed on them, but the poor sick civilians had had none; they were regarded as intruders. Amongst them were Maltese, Greeks, Italians, Americans, Germans, and Negroes. Some of the Russian prisoners were there also. Without neglecting the soldiers, we were able to show some special attention to these poor fellows. Strangers in a foreign land, they had the greatest claim to compassion.

All were at work, and on our very first day we had visits from some of our Scutari and Koulali friends. Father Unsworth, an extremely nice English priest, and the senior chaplain in the Crimea, was also a visitor. Nothing, he said, could be more edifying than to see Lord Killeen going at the head of his gallant hussars so punctually to Mass on Sundays—five hundred cavalry, with their brass helmets and long swords, mounted on their chargers, ascending the great hills to pay homage to the God of Armies.

Sister M. Elizabeth's brother, Captain Hersey, a young officer of only twenty, came to visit her, dressed in his uniform (within the last few years this gentleman built a church at his own expense in Galway for the use of the soldiers). Young lads of seventeen and eighteen were being sent out to fill the ranks. From a hill at the back of our hut we had a view of the English, French, Sardinian, and Turkish camps.

CHAPTER 8

Two Martyrs of Mercy

Each Sister had charge of two wards, and there was just at this time a fresh outbreak of cholera. The Sisters were up every night; and the cases, as in Scutari and Koulali, were nearly all fatal. Rev. Mother did not allow the Sisters to remain up at night, except in cases of cholera, without a written order from the doctor.

In passing to the wards at night we used to meet the rats in droves. They would not even move out of our way. They were there before us, and were determined to keep possession. As for our own hut, they evidently wanted to make it theirs, scraping under the boards, jumping up on the shelf where our little tin utensils were kept, rattling everything. One night, dear Sister M. Paula found one licking her forehead she had a real horror of them. Sleep was out of the question. Our third day in Balaklava was a very sad one for us. One of our dear band, Sister Winifred, got very ill during the night with cholera. She was a most angelic Sister, and we were all deeply grieved.

She was attacked, at about three o'clock in the morning, with the symptoms which were now so well known to us: every remedy was applied; our beloved Rev. Mother never left her; she was attended by Father Unsworth, from whom she received the last rites of our holy religion; and she calmly breathed her last on the evening of the same day. A hut was arranged in which to place the remains; and, so alarming were the rats—and such huge animals were they—that we had to watch during the night, so that they should not touch her.

She, the first to go of our little band, had been full of life and energy the day before. We were all very sad, and we wondered who would be the next. Rev. Mother was anxious to have her buried near Father Wheble, the first Crimean Martyr. But Sir John Hall said that that place was likely to be desecrated, and that it was better to look elsewhere. And they did, indeed, find on the hills of Balaklava a spot of ground between two rocks, with just room for about two graves, and this was her last resting-place.

Father Woollett, Father Unsworth, and Father Malony preceded the coffin chanting the prayers, and we followed immediately after. Miss Nightingale was at the funeral, and even joined in the prayers. The soldiers, doctors, officers, and officials followed. When all was over, we returned to our hut, very sad; but we had no further time to think. Patients were pouring in, and we should be out again to the cholera wards. Besides cholera, there were cases of fever, in fact of every disease. Others had been nearly killed by the blasting of rocks, and they came in fearfully disfigured.

Father Woollett brought us one day a present of a Russian cat; he bought it, he told us, from an old Russian woman, for the small sum of seven shillings. It made a particularly handsome captive in the land of its fathers; for we were obliged to keep it tied to a chair, to prevent its escape. But the very sight of this powerful champion soon relieved us of some of our unwelcome and voracious visitors. The arrival of Father Duffy, S.J., from Dublin, did something to cheer us up at this time. Also, an officer waited on Rev. Mother to say that the men of his regiment, the 89th, begged as a favour that they might be allowed to put a marble cross over Sister Winifred's grave. She did not hesitate to accept with gratitude this mark of kindness.

The extra kitchen got on well—a stone building, with a large oven like a baker's. I do not know if it was there before the English arrived, or was built purposely. At all events, it suited very well; we had a charcoal stove also; the dinner tins were placed all round this to keep everything hot. I had the charge of this, helped by three first-class orderlies, besides a party of what are called fatigue men, who came down every day from the "Front." To have everything served hot and comfortable to the different wards was our dearest Mother's earnest wish, and many a lecture had the Sister-in-charge on the subject rice, sago, arrowroot, chops when they could be got, and sometimes chickens.

If the orderlies had their own way, they would wring the head off the chicken, put it down with the feathers on, and then take off the skin and feathers together; they thought we gave ourselves entirely too much trouble. They used to take great pleasure in having the kitchen very clean. One morning, when I went to see after the breakfast, I said: "Really, Tom, the kitchen is beautifully clean."

"Yes, Ma'am, he replied, "and we have the milk made as well."

A great piece of shell came down one day, and made a terrific noise at the kitchen door.

I really got a fright, and said, "Oh, are the Russians coming?"

"No, Ma'am," said one of my orderlies, "and if they are itself, many a fine British soldier will be laid low before one of ye are touched."

There were many useful things in the stores suitable for the kitchen, but it was next to impossible to get anything out of them. You would be told over and over that there was not such a thing to be had. But Rev. Mother was all energy where the wants of the sick were concerned, and made a great fight with Mr. Fitzgerald, the Deputy-Purveyor, till she got what she wanted. Mr. Scott-Robinson sent us waterproof cloaks from Constantinople at this time. There was rain and snow, and he thought we might find them useful; but they were of too fine and delicate a texture for us. They were French, and only fit for French ladies. We returned them with many thanks.

Rumours of peace came one day only to be contradicted the next. Rev. Mother now received a letter from Dr. Lyons (son of Sir W. Lyons, of Cork), who wanted to know if there was anything he could do for us. He was stationed at the "Front," and he advised her to get out more nuns, as they were sure to be wanted. Other hospitals, he said, were to be opened, and who could do the work like the nuns? I hope we did not get proud.

Christmas had come round once more. It was fearfully cold—the soldiers said that the wind blowing from Sebastopol would cut the head off a man. That Christmas Day of 1855 we had four Masses, and crowds at Holy Communion. We had a saintly chaplain, Father Gleeson, a Vincentian. He had no mercy on himself. He came out with a little stuff soutane and not a particle of warm clothing.

We could only hope that when our little Jesuit, Father Woollett, came from the camp he would make him put on a suit of fur like his own. Rev. Mother gave him warm gloves and a muffler, but he came down next morning without them. She gave him a great scolding, but it was all the same. The climate was so fickle that, after a sunny day our blankets might be frozen at night.

There was great work in the kitchen that Christmas Day. There were any number of nice puddings, and even plum puddings for the orderlies, who had a little money to spare and procured what was necessary for them. But only imagine, the rats, the dreadful rats, sucked a hundred eggs in the night, and killed the few chickens that were for the day. We were all indignant—and the eggs so scarce too. What was to be done? Well, the best we could, and the puddings were not too bad.

We had a good deal of cleaning up in the kitchen after the Christmas dinner, and our fatigue men were from the cavalry regiments: they looked so respectable I often felt a little delicate at asking them to do any dirty work. An officer came every evening to collect his men, and he generally said: "I hope, Sister, you have no complaint to make." We never had any. Very often these men had to go the same night to the trenches, or other places of danger.

At this date a friend in the camp sent Rev. Mother a copy of *The Illustrated London News*, with the following paragraph:

> Miss Wise has been succeeded by sixteen nuns (we were only fifteen), principally Irish ladies, who, having received instructions from Miss Nightingale, appear to be very attentive to their charge, and eminently deserving the name they bear—Sisters of Mercy. They are attired from head to foot in the deepest black; even their heads are carefully hooded. The only relief to this sombre attire is the double string of beads hanging from their girdles. I was quite startled on my first introduction to one of these ladies. I had not even heard of their arrival, and, having a patient in a very critical state in one of the hospital huts, I went down about midnight to pay him a visit. On opening the door, I beheld by the light of a wretched little lamp just such a phantom as Bulwer has drawn in *Lucretia*: darkness in every corner of the room, and a tall figure draped and hooded—darker even than the night—gliding from bed to bed. I am sorry to say that one of the Sisters, two days after their arrival, was seized with cholera and died.

During the month of January fever cases became very numerous, and, of course, night watching continuous. If a fever patient is not well nursed during the night no amount of care will bring back what he loses—some nourishment must be given every two hours, or more frequently, as the doctor may direct; we had bad cases of typhus and typhoid, and in these cases, nursing is everything. The doctors were often surprised in the morning to find their patients so well over the night—no matter how clever a doctor may be, if he has not a good nurse, who will attend strictly to his directions, little can be done. The following report, sent by the Deputy-Purveyor to the War Office, dated December 24th, 1855, came before me only lately, and I hope it will not be out of place here. He says:

> The superiority of an ordered system is beautifully illustrated in the Sisters of Mercy. One mind appears to move all, and their intelligence, delicacy, and conscientiousness invest them with a halo of extreme confidence. The medical officer can safely consign his most critical cases to their hands. Stimulants or opiates ordered every five minutes will be faithfully administered though the five minutes' labour were repeated uninterruptedly for a week. The number of Sisters, without being large, is sufficient to secure for every patient needing it his share of attention: a calm resigned contentedness sits on the features of all, and the soft cares of the woman and the lady breathe placidly throughout.

The Sisters engaged in the wards found it a great help to have the extra kitchen carefully attended to. Though the orderlies were good and fairly sober, still they could not be trusted in preparing food in any way fit for a delicate patient—it could scarcely be expected. Whenever they went to the "Front," to get their pay, no matter what good resolutions they made, they were very seldom presentable for a day or two.

Early in 1856 rumours of peace reached us from all sides. But our Heavenly Father demanded another sacrifice from our devoted little band. Dear Sister Mary Elizabeth was called to a Martyr's crown.

She was specially beloved for her extraordinary sweetness of disposition. The doctor, when called, pronounced her illness to be fever—she had caught typhus in her ward. Every loving care was bestowed on her by our dearest Mother, who scarcely ever left her bedside. Death seemed to have no sting for this saintly Religious—she was continually renewing her vows and making her profession of faith. She had no wish to live or die, feeling she was in the arms of her Heavenly Father. "He will do for me what is best," she whispered, "and His will is all I desire."

A little before her death she said: "Rev. Mother, I could never express to you how happy I feel. There is not one drawback."

Rev. Mother said to her: "You know, dear Sister, all our wants. Will you not help us when you see God face to face?"

"Oh, yes," she said, "I surely will." She thanked all the Sisters, embraced and took leave of them most affectionately, retaining her senses to the very last. She had no agony—the fever simply consumed her.

It was a wild, wild night. The storm and wind penetrated the chinks so as to extinguish the lights, and evoked many a prayer that the death-bed might not be left roofless. It was awful beyond description to kneel beside her during these hours of her passage and to hear the solemn prayers for the dead and dying mingled with the howling of the winds and the creaking of the frail wooden hut. Oh, never, never can any of us forget that night: the storm disturbed all but her, that happy being or whom earth's joys and sorrows were at an end, and whose summons home had not cost her one pang or one regret. Her happy death occurred on Saturday, the 23rd of February.

The death of our dear Sister Mary Elizabeth was announced by the chaplain in the different divisions after Mass. It was also announced that the office would be at three, and the funeral immediately after. The 89th begged Father Unsworth to ask the captain to allow them off parade, that they might attend the funeral, which he willingly did. Detachments from every regiment joined them. The 89th requested the honour of being allowed to carry the coffin. Hundreds of soldiers formed a treble file on each side of the passage from the hospital to the hut, where eight priests, the Sisters, and the soldiers chosen to bear the coffin had assembled.

Every head was uncovered as the procession passed slowly down the hill to the chapel. It was a thrilling sight to see the multitude of various nations, ranks, and employments, amid holy silence unbroken save by the voice of tearful supplication. A contest arose later between the medical staff and the officers as to which should have the honour of putting a cross on her grave. We took no part, save to feel truly grateful for the kind feeling of which it was evidence.

The graves of our two dear Sisters were tended with loving kindness. A chaplain who visited the place long after the Sisters had left, found these lonely graves on the brow of that rugged hill enclosed by a high iron railing set in cut stone—the whole being visible from the Black Sea beneath. They were decked with beautiful flowers and evergreens planted by the loving hands of their soldier friends, and marked with white marble crosses bearing their simple epitaph. On the arm of the cross of Sister Winifred's grave the priest found a paper, on which were written the following lines, composed, as he afterwards heard, by one of her orderlies:

Still green be the willow that grows on the mountain,
And weeps o'er the grave of the Sister that's gone;

✶✶✶✶✶✶

And most glorious its lot to point out to the stranger,
The hallowed remains of the sainted and blest;
For those angels of mercy had dared every danger,
To bring to the soldier sweet comfort and rest.

Some other verses, these written by a friend, on the death of Sister Winifred, may be allowed a place in this history:

They laid her in her lonely grave upon a foreign strand,
Far from her own dear island home, far from her native land.
They bore her to her long last home amid the clash of arms,
And the hymn they sang seemed sadly sweet amid war's fierce alarms.

They heeded not the cannon's roar, the rifle's deadly shot,
But onward still they sadly went to gain that lowly spot;
And there, with many a fervent prayer and many a word of love,
They left her in her lowly grave with a simple cross above.

And yet she was a gentle soul, a timid fearful thing,
Who, like a startled fawn, had sought her Convent's shelt'ring wing;
Had left with glad and bounding heart a world she could not love,
And chosen for her own chaste spouse the Lamb of stainless love.

She thought to spend her peaceful days within those cloisters grey,
And with Matin song and Vesper hymn beguile her life away.
She little thought again to roam amid the world's dark strife,
Save where sweet mercy led her steps to soothe the woes of life.

Yet far away from her Convent grey, and far from her lowly cell,
And far from the soft and silvery tone of the sweet Convent bell,
And far from the home she loved so well, and far from her native sky,
'Mid the cannon's roar on a hostile shore she laid her down to die.

She loved full well her Convent home, and loved its cloisters grey,
And loved full well those holy spots where she had knelt to pray,
Yet, with a purer, deeper love, she loved the soldier brave,
And left her home, and left her all, his sinking soul to save.

She went not forth to gain applause, she sought not empty fame;
E'en those she tended might not know her history or her name;
No honours waited on her path, no flattering voice was nigh;
For she only sought to toil and love, and mid her toil to die.

They raise no trophy to her name, they rear no stately bust,
To tell the stranger where she rests, co-mingling with the dust;
They leave her in her lowly grave, beneath that foreign sky,

Where she had taught them how to live, and taught them how to die.

Sister Winifred was English by birth, and Sister Elizabeth was Irish.

Chapter 9
In and Out of Combat

About this time fresh accusations were made to the War Office, to the commander-in-chief, and others, that the Sisters interfered in religious matters with the non-Catholic patients. It became so serious that Rev. Mother wrote to Lord Raglan, explaining the strictly conscientious attitude of the Sisters. His Lordship expressed himself pleased and satisfied; indeed, no one could hold intercourse with our beloved Mother M. F. Bridgeman without recognising in her the highest form of principle and practice. She had given her word not to interfere with the religion of non-Catholic patients, and, rather than violate that word, as everyone who knew her felt, she would willingly undergo any martyrdom.

There was no danger of her violating her contract, even when attempts were made to encroach on her own rights. It is quite clear that our dear Mother had much to endure from these continual false accusations, not one of which was even attempted to be proved against us.

And all this time we did not, I believe, get even a shirt, a pair of stockings, in fact any article of clothing, from the stores; but we had tracts reviling our holy religion, as well as pictures of the worst description, too bad to be written about—the writer of this sketch pleads guilty to having burned thousands of them, and in doing so believes she was doing good for the Protestant soldiers as much as the Catholic. In the midst of all this we had many kind friends. Protestants were quite as ready to defend us as Catholics. Lord Napier and Ettrick frequently bore testimony to the fidelity with which the nuns kept to their contract of non-interference. At Edinburgh, on a later occasion, he said:

> At an early period of my life I held a diplomatic position under Lord Stratford de Redcliffe, in Constantinople. During the distress of the Crimean War the ambassador called me one morning and said: 'Go down to the port; you will find a ship there loaded with Jewish exiles—Russian subjects from the Crimea. It is your duty to disembark them. The Turks will give you a house in which they may be placed. I turn them over entirely

to you.'

I went down to the shore and received about two hundred persons, the most miserable objects that could be witnessed, most of them old men, women, and children. I placed them in the cold, ruinous lodging allocated to them by the Ottoman authorities. I went back to the ambassador, and said: 'Your Excellency, these people are cold, and I have no fuel or blankets. They are hungry, and I have no food. They are dirty, and I have no soap. Their hair is in an indescribable condition, and I have no combs. What am I to do with these people?'

'Do?' said the ambassador. 'Get a couple of Sisters of Mercy, they will put all to right in a moment.'

I went, saw the Mother Superior, and explained the case. I asked for two Sisters. She ordered two from her presence to follow me. They were ladies of refinement and intellect. I was a stranger and a Protestant, and I invoked their assistance for the benefit of Jews. Yet these two women made up their bundles and followed me through the rain, without a look, a whisper, a sign of hesitation. From that moment my fugitives were saved. I witnessed the labours of those Sisters for months, and they never endeavoured to make a single convert.

The military men were not less enthusiastic. When Colonel Connolly, brother-in-law to Mr. Bruin, of Carlow, was travelling, after his return from the war, near the Bruin Estate, a fellow-traveller spoke disrespectfully of nuns. The colonel, a Protestant, not only made a warm defence of the ladies who had nursed him in Russian and Ottoman regions, and for their sakes of all other nuns, but handed the assailant his card, saying: "If you say another word against these saintly gentlewomen I shall call you out." The slanderer subsided very quickly.

It was said at one time that the War Office was on the point of issuing a mandate forbidding us to speak even to the Catholic soldiers on religion—or to say a prayer for them. However, that mandate never came: we often thought the Guardian Angels of the soldiers prevented it. Dear Rev. Mother wrote to her own bishop, telling him of our troubles, and the following was his reply:

My dear Rev. Mother,

Your work is so manifestly the work of God that we must expect various contradictions as a matter of course. Whatever they may be there is always one even course to be followed: bear up cheerfully and happily against them all, be firm in your just rule of acting, and do not leave your post. It is only when you have returned to your native home, full of merit before God, that you can begin to enjoy fully the happiness of your present mission. The works you are engaged in would in themselves seem of sufficient importance to justify all the labours you have endured and all the risks you have encountered.

It is scarcely necessary for me to say anything in confirmation of the duties and calling of a Sister of Mercy. Noble as benevolence undoubtedly is, you are not mere philanthropists in the restricted meaning of the term, though in its true sense the philanthropist is one who would minister to the comfort, the true and great comfort of the soul no less than to the wants of the body. I thank God most fervently for the manifest protection afforded you in your many trials, and hope to see all return home soon and happily. I remain, dear Rev. Mother,

With sincere regard, yours very truly,

William Delany.

We had received also the following letter from Dr. Manning—afterwards Cardinal—in allusion to the many trials with which our path was likely to be strewn:

78 South Audley Street, December 1st, 1854.

My dear Sisters in Jesus Christ,

It seems but right that a few words of encouragement should be addressed to you who have so generously offered yourselves to go on a new and difficult mission, in which many unusual and unforeseen trials may come upon you. You will, however, always bear in mind for whose sake you go forth, and to whom your services of consolation are rendered. This thought, without such words at least as I can write, will suffice to strengthen and to cheer you under all you may have to endure. Nevertheless, there are certain points on which you may not think a few words without their use.

At first, you may perhaps meet with many privations and inconveniences in leaving the quiet and order of your simple Convent home to enter on a life of travel, activity, and labour, sometimes it may be with slender or bad provisions for food and dwelling, and with rough fare, even in the few things your ordinary life requires.

You will not, I know, let privations or hardships overcome you or draw from you a word of complaining; but you will bear all those things with a cheerful heart for His sake Who often had not so much as time to eat, nor had He where to lay His head. Again, in conversing with many people, as you needs must do, you cannot fail to meet with many trials from the ill temper of the evil, the slights and injustice of adversaries, the rudeness and censure of many who are good in many ways.

Prepare yourselves for this mortification, and offer it gladly to our Divine Lord, who bore all manner of contradiction for you. Another subject about which you will have need to exercise yourselves in the spirit of patient and glad compliance will be the work of learning how to treat medical and surgical cases. All of you have probably had experience in nursing ordinary sickness, and that alone is enough to make you feel how much more will be required of you than you have yet had opportunity to learn: you are going, therefore, to work as learners with a spirit of exactness and humility, and you will receive,

I well know, the directions of physicians and surgeons with a prompt and cheerful readiness. We need never be ashamed to learn, and every lesson we acquire is a new gift—which we may lay out again in the service of Our Lord. Begin your work, therefore, from the beginning, from the simplest rules of practice, and learn accurately everything which relates to the care of the sick, the dressing of wounds, the handling of special cases of medical or surgical treatment. Being already called to the grace of the more perfect life, be not content with an imperfect or ordinary knowledge and skill in the nursing of the sick and wounded, but strive to be as perfect in this ministry of consolation as in the life of the counsels.

And, lastly, be not discouraged at the change from the recollection and tranquillity of your cloister and choir to the ceaseless motion and publicity of the world of work, in which you will have to live. God is able to make the hospital a cloister and your own heart a choir. His graces will be with you in the measure of your daily and hourly need. If you leave Him in the silence of your Convent it is to find Him by the bedside of the wounded. You leave Christ, for Christ, and wheresoever you go for His sake He will be with you.

Many prayers will be put up for you without ceasing, and of-

tentimes the Holy Sacrifice will be offered for you that you may "spend and be spent" with glad hearts for our dear Lord's sake, and receive from Him the reward of joy which is laid up for those who serve Him in the least of his brethren. May His loving care bring you safely home again; if not, I trust there will be more crowns in Heaven. Forgive these words from one who has no worthiness to be your counsellor, and give me a place in your prayers; and may the grace of God be with you all! Believe me, my dear Sisters in Christ, Your faithful and humble servant
for His sake,

Henry Edward Manning.

By degrees patients became less numerous, and news was continually reaching us that peace was certain. However, the doctors wished us to remain till the last, and Rev. Mother would have done so but for an unexpected event.

Before we came to Balaklava in October, Miss Nightingale had withdrawn her nurses, so that the hospital was vacant. Now, Miss Nightingale was named by the War Office as the Superintendent of the nursing staff in the East; and in April, 1856, she again assumed the charge of the General Hospital at Balaklava, saying she had directions from the War Office to do so. Under these circumstances, and as peace was being proclaimed, Rev. Mother made up her mind to leave. The patients were nearly all convalescent; and she was rather glad to get home before the great crush of soldiers and civilians started for England. Miss Nightingale was very anxious that we should remain. However, Rev. Mother thought it was not necessary, and wrote the following letter to Sir John Hall:

Dear Sir,
As it is no longer in your power to continue us here on the terms on which you accepted our services in the Crimea, I beg to resign my charge to you from whom I have received it. May I also offer my best thanks for the uniform kindness we have received from you and those who represent you? For it, as well as for the cordial cooperation and appreciation shown us, we shall ever feel grateful. During the sixteen months of our Mission in the East, our difficulties and trials have been many, and often painful and perplexing. But it is due to the medical officers, as well as to those of the Purveying Department, to say

that they did not arise from them—these we have found ever willing to work with us and kindly and cordially to accept our services. Then, the delicate and cautious respect and gratitude ever evinced by the patients of different creeds and countries has been to us a source of constant thankfulness. May I beg you will kindly take the necessary means to arrange for our passage home as soon as convenient? and

Believe me to be, dear Sir,
Yours faithfully in Jesus Christ,
Sister M. F. Bridgeman.

This is what Sir John Hall wrote in reply:

My dear Madam,
I cannot permit you and the Sisters under your direction to leave the Crimea without an expression of the high opinion I entertain of your administration, and of the very important aid you have rendered to the sick under your care. I can most conscientiously assert, as I have on other occasions stated, that you have given me the most perfect satisfaction ever since you assumed the charge of the nursing department of the General Hospital at Balaklava, and I do most unfeignedly regret your departure. But, after what has occurred I would not, even with that feeling uppermost in my mind, urge you to stay.
I enclose a letter from Sir William Codrington, Commander-in-Chief, expressive of the sense he entertains of your services and those of the Sisters, which I trust will be acceptable to your feelings; and I feel assured you must leave us with an approving conscience, as I know you do with the blessings of those you have aided in their hour of need. To Him Who sees all our outward actions, and knows our inmost thoughts and wishes, I commend you. And may He have you and those with you in His holy keeping is the prayer of yours faithfully,

John Hall, Inspector-General of Hospitals.

This distinguished medical officer often recalled with pleasure his connection with the Sisters of Mercy in the East, and continued to take the deepest interest in their Institute. Once, when some postulants for the Sisters of Mercy happened to be in the same vessel with him, going to New Zealand, he no sooner learned their destination than he took them, as it were, under his protection—paid them the most polite and fatherly attention, taught them little games, and did all he could to relieve the monotony of their voyage. But, above all, he awakened their enthusiasm by speaking of his acquaintance with the Sisters in the Eastern hospitals, giving instances of their bearing during those perilous times.

The following was the letter from Sir William Codrington to Sir John Hall:

Sir,

I regret much to hear that circumstances have induced Mrs. Bridgeman, Superior of the Roman Catholic Sisters, to quit the General Hospital and proceed to England with the Sisters who have been associated with her. I request you to assure that lady of the high estimation in which her services and those of the Sisters are held by us all, founded as that opinion is on the experience of yourself, the medical officer of the hospitals, and of the many patients, both wounded and sick, who, during the fourteen or fifteen months past, have benefited by their care. I am quite sure that their unfailing kindness will have the reward which Mrs. Bridgeman values, viz., the remembrance and gratitude of those who have been the objects of such disinterested attention.—Your obedient servant,

W. Codrington, General Commander.

These have paid their tribute to our Rev. Mother—I will pay mine. That she was richly endowed with gifts of nature and grace was beyond all doubt. Her very appearance, her manner, and address, were most attractive, and her mind and talents highly cultivated. But, above all, there was a halo of sanctity about her that seemed to have entwined the affections of those who knew her closely around her. The Sisters she had in the East were from different Communities: some from Dublin, Carlow, Cork, Kinsale, Charleville, Liverpool, and Chelsea.

Yet one and all of them held her in the same love and veneration—and with all these superior talents she governed more like a Sister than a Superior. We used to gather round her in the evenings, and tell her all the events of the day. She had many sleepless nights, but they were spent in prayer, in close commune with Him for Whom she lived and laboured. I could wish every word I have said to be written in letters of gold; and, perhaps, there were few of the Sisters who knew her better than I did. Her whole anxiety was that we should keep alive the interior spirit, and be as much Religious in our new sphere of action as in our Convent homes. Some of her "beautiful reminders," as we used to call them, are noted in our old journals.

Though our Sisters from Bermondsey were with Miss Nightingale at the Barrack Hospital, we rarely met— it was such an enormous place, capable of accommodating some thousands of soldiers. They left England with her, and of them she speaks most affectionately.

CHAPTER 10

Homeward Bound

When we began our work of packing up and preparing for the voyage, we had many visitors. Miss Nightingale, the Protestant clergyman of Koulali, Dr. Beatsin, Dr. Hamilton (of the Guards), the Purveyor, Father Unsworth, Father Duffy, S.J., Father Strickland, S.J., and poor soldiers and orderlies in crowds.

We sailed from Balaklava on the 12th of April: the day was beautifully fine, and the accommodation in the *Cleopatra* first class. We owed an everlasting debt of gratitude to Sir John Hall, for his great kindness in thus arranging for our homeward voyage. We had a private saloon; the captain told us he had got orders to see after our comfort in every way; and Father Woollett, S.J., accompanied us.

A two days' sail across the Black Sea brought us in view of the minarets and mosques of Constantinople, with the beautiful marble palace of its *Sultan*. We anchored in the Bosphorus for a day or two, and had visits from the Sisters of Charity, priests, doctors, and other kind friends. We had a lovely view from the vessel, and gave a last sad look at the once beautiful Church of Santa Sophia, now, alas! a Turkish mosque; a church once so magnificent that, when the Emperor Justinian entered it after it was completed, he exclaimed in an ecstasy of delight: "Solomon, I have surpassed thee." It was the most richly decorated temple that ever stood upon the earth. The altar was solid gold encrusted with the most precious and costly stones. There, also, St. Gregory the Great and St. John Chrysostom preached and laboured.

As the vessel moved, we took a last look at gorgeous Constantinople. The Russians call it the city of the *Czar*—time will tell that, I suppose. We passed Therapia and our former hospital, Koulali. Soon all the beauteous sights were lost to our view; we sailed into the Dardanelles and arrived at Gallipoli. As we sailed through the Archipelago, we passed Abydos. We reached Malta that evening—*Deo gratias*. Three or four rockets were let off and two blue lights; the pilot arrived and we were soon in the harbour. The admiral's boat drew up, and an officer stepped on board to make official inquiries—whence we came, whither we went, and who or what the main body on board were.

Having been answered satisfactorily, the happy official went his way. A cannon-shot from a man-of-war lying near us announced the hour of nine, and we were off to rest. At half-past six in the morning two Jesuits came on board to convey us over in a boat. The Maltese who rowed the boat took out their scapulars and put them outside their jackets, that we might know they belonged to us. It was a most delightful morning. We got Mass, confession, and Holy Communion at the famous Church of the Knights of St. John: the Jesuits had no church of their own in Malta, but officiated at St. John's.

When we had finished our thanksgiving, we were conducted by Father Woollett and another kind Father to their college, where we had the privilege of sharing the hospitality of the good Fathers. There is a beautiful throne inside the sanctuary, near the stalls once occupied by the knights. We heard this was erected for the use of Mr. Moore O'Ferrall, who was Governor there for some time. But we were told he never used it, preferring to kneel and pray amongst the poor people. *"The prayers of the humble shall pierce the clouds."* Our vessel was waiting for us, and we could make no further delay. The morning of the 30th brought us in view of the rock of Gibraltar, and we arrived there at noon.

The Most Rev. Dr. Hughes and many priests came to visit us. The bishop thought we should go to his palace, and had his carriage waiting for us: but as we did not go, he remained with us nearly all day. He was Irish, thoroughly Irish; he wore a large black cloak and a broad brimmed hat with a piece of green ribbon around it: we often heard of him from the soldiers who were stationed at Malta; they all seemed to know and love him. The day was fine, and we were all on deck, so we gathered round him to hear his beautiful stories.

It was now the 1st of May, and Ascension Day. We set sail again, and passed Cape St. Vincent. Our passengers were few. One was Major Pakenham, a distinguished hero of Alma and cousin to the victor of Waterloo. We were greatly amused when he told us he had with difficulty got into the ship, the captain of which assured him he had got orders to keep things very quiet for the nuns. The major said he would neither sing nor dance! We became great friends. He was most anxious to know how we spent our evenings; he said he knew very well how we spent the day.

He was quite delighted when he heard we had such happy, cheerful evenings, and could play, sing, or do anything that gave us pleasure. He spoke with respect and affection of his cousin, the Hon. Charles Pakenham, once a captain in the Guards, who, exchanging a sword of steel for the sword of the spirit, was received into the Church by Cardinal Wiseman, and became a Passionist Father.

The wind was in our favour, and at last we approached the dreaded Bay of Biscay. But our voyage was, on the whole, a good one. In the English Channel we had rather a cold and dreary reception. On the 7th of May we came in sight of land, and hoped to be in Spithead that evening. We soon after arrived at Portsmouth, and after much railroad fuss we started for London, accompanied by Father Woollett, S.J. We reached the London terminus at about nine, and went to Blandford Square Convent, where thousands of loving greetings awaited us.

After a delay of two days, during which time we visited our much-loved Sisters at Chelsea, and had innumerable visitors, including Cardinal Wiseman, came the dreaded parting with our much loved Mother M. F. Bridgeman and her two Kinsale Sisters—she having determined to visit her convent in Derby.

That parting left a blank in each heart never to be filled up till the last trumpet will bring us all and our cherished friends together to that happy home where partings and sorrows are unknown.

We left Blandford Square for our convent in Liverpool, and we spent two happy days there. The Dublin, Carlow, Cork, and Charleville Sisters arrived in Baggot Street on the morning of *Corpus Christi*, 1856. A grand *Te Deum* was sung after Mass, and no Sisters of Mercy ever got a more loving welcome than we got from our dear Sisters at Baggot Street. Then we all looked anxiously to our own Convent homes. Some started next day, and others had to remain to see one or other, and amongst the rest the Carlow Sisters. The archbishop was out of town, and left word for us to wait till his return; but our dear friend, Dr. Dunne, came when he heard we had arrived, and told us it was better to start at once by the evening train, that great preparations were being made in the town to give us a reception, and that we were not expected till next day. We were only too glad to start at once.

Arrived in Carlow, we got down to the Convent quickly, but not without cheers for the "Russian Nuns." The dear Sisters we parted from eighteen months before were all inside the gate to welcome us. When the bishop heard of our arrival, he sent Dean Hughes to bid us welcome, and say that he would come himself in the morning, and that there would be a solemn High Mass of Thanksgiving for our safe return on the following Sunday, in the cathedral, to conclude with the *Te Deum*.

CHAPTER 11
After Many Days

At the urgent request of some respected friends, I have embodied in the foregoing pages the substance of my old Crimean journal which has been so long thrown aside. Our much-loved Rev. Mother M. F. Bridgeman and all the Sisters have gone to their eternal home, save one, the writer of this journal, the most unworthy of the cherished band. But their labours did not end with that eventful mission. In the service of the suffering poor, in hospitals, schools, and orphanages, and in visiting them in their wretched homes, they worked bravely on to the end, till their heavenly Bridegroom called them to receive the reward of their hidden labours.

This *journal* would be much more interesting could I have seen each little diary kept by the dear Sisters who are gone; but they have nearly all disappeared except one, and my own was in great part eaten by the rats at Balaklava. Carlow was my first Convent home; from there I went to the East, and soon after my return I was sent to Gort, county Galway, where I now am.

If any of the English ladies or others who have aided in the mission are still alive, I beg to send them my warmest remembrance, and an assurance that I have daily remembered them in my unworthy prayers. Of one of these ladies, I may add a word. Soon after Rev. Mother's return to Kinsale, Cardinal Wiseman sent her the following letter which he had received, and which he thought would give her pleasure:

My Lord Cardinal,
Casually taking up the *Record* of the 4th inst., the following words arrested my attention—they form part of an extract of a "*Lenten Indult*" read in Roman Catholic churches, and which purports to emanate from yourself: "Circumstances seemed to call upon them to pay a public tribute to a class of labourers in the Aceldama of the Crimea—their humble but laborious nuns. It must have been a source of pain to Roman Catholics that no manifestation of feeling had ever been witnessed towards them, while charity that had sprung up suddenly in the world had

been honoured by Royal praise, and commemorated by lasting monuments."

Of the labours of the Sisters of Mercy in the Crimea it is not for me to speak. I know of them only by report of those who witnessed them, and thankfully bear testimony to their priceless value; but of the twelve nuns who worked at Balaklava, eight were under my direction at Koulali from the 10th of April to October 1st, 1855. I consider it a privilege to bear witness to their devotion and obedience, to the perfect truthfulness and exquisite tact with which they performed the duties of nursing during those weary months.

As an individual, my testimony is of little value; but the position which I then occupied gave me opportunity which no other possessed of watching—and I did so narrowly—the spirit which guided them, and the manner in which their work was done; and rather than the deep injustice of refusing all honour and thanks to the Roman Catholic Sisters of Mercy should be done in England's name, I have broken the silence most dear and fitting to a woman. Much more might be said; but I know that neither the Mother Frances or her Sisters seek for praise here, and, at the risk of exciting a smile at Protestant fondness for Scriptural allusion, I would add that they are surely blessed in not receiving their reward of men.—I am, my Lord Cardinal, yours faithfully,

Emily Hutton,
Lady Superintendent at Koulali Hospital.

Father Strickland died in the Crimea, where he caught typhus fever in the French Hospital. He was buried with such military honours as usually accompany to the grave only a general officer of the first rank. Father Strickland was generally beloved and respected in the camp. When fever and scurvy raged like a plague amongst the French troops—many of the French chaplains fell victims—the men were daily dying without Sacrament.

The three Jesuits, Father Woollett, Father Duffy, and Father Strickland, offered their aid, as there was very little sick duty amongst the English troops; and they daily rode over to the French, and spent a portion of each day in their hospitals. Father Woollett first caught fever, but recovered; Father Strickland went to an early grave, and is now, I trust, enjoying a martyr's crown, the fruit of his zeal and charity—the sixth priest buried in the Crimea.

In December, 1856, the convents heard that Bishop Grant had been officially informed that the *Sultan* graciously wished to present the Sisters who had nursed the Turks as well as Christians in the Ottoman Empire with a memento of his appreciation of their services. Lord Panmure, in making this communication, besought the bishop to express to the "Sisterhood the sense entertained by Her Majesty's Government of the devotion displayed by them in attending and mitigating the sufferings of the sick and wounded soldiers in the East."

The nuns, whose services had been wholly gratuitous, declined to accept any gift which might be construed as a remuneration; but as a decided refusal might be offensive to a foreign Potentate, whose expressed appreciation of their services was entirely unexpected, they laid the matter before authority. The following was Cardinal Wiseman's reply to the Mother Superior of the Carlow House:

London, December 17th, 1856.

My dear Cousin and Rev. Mother,

After mature consideration I decided that the nuns of Bermondsey, on their coming to our hospital, should accept the *Sultan's* gift, it being quite understood by the War Office that it was not bestowed on the individual nuns, but on pious works through the hands of their communities. This being the case, why refuse to accept a sum, however small, for the poor, which, if refused, will only go to Protestants for worldly purposes? I own I do not see why.

In Ireland there may be reasons which I do not know, but here there are not. I could not consistently allow or advise one house to accept and tell another to refuse. I must, therefore, reply to your note that I think you should accept and apply the money to some charitable purpose.—Your affectionate cousin and Father in Christ,

N. Card. Wiseman.

Bishop Grant wrote to Cardinal Cullen on the same subject; and other letters that followed may be given here:

December 15th, 1856.

My Lord Archbishop,

The War Office has taken great pains to arrange the *Sultan's* gift in the way least likely for the nuns to receive it. They told me to write the accompanying letter, which was to express that the

Sisters received it for distribution amongst the poor, and in no way for themselves; and I am glad that Your Grace has seen no difficulty in allowing the Baggot Street Community to receive it. The Sisters of Mercy in other Convents in Ireland objected, but I think that the enclosed letter guards them sufficiently, especially when it is considered that they have received no communication from our own Government, and they remain, therefore, as they were, free from any gift or reward. If Your Grace approves, will you represent this to the Bishop of Kildare and Leighlin, so that his Sisters may not object to receive the gift.—Yours sincerely,

Thomas Grant.

To Sir B. Hawes.

The revised list of the Sisters of Mercy who attended the hospitals in the East are now in your hands, and in the name of their respective Communities I beg leave to express their gratitude to the Government for having allowed them to assist their brave fellow countrymen during the war.

It is pleasing to them to reflect that their desire to undertake the duties assigned them solely from motives of charity and without any personal remuneration has been admitted and recognised by their country; and that, therefore, in being permitted to distribute the gift of His Imperial Majesty the *Sultan* amongst the poor and infirm, they will not lose the honour which they so highly prized of having been allowed to devote their services, without hope of any earthly reward, to the alleviation of the sufferings and care of the sick and dying soldiers of the expeditionary army. If you still intend me to receive the gift of the *Sultan*, it will be my duty to forward the letters to the respective Communities to whom it is sent, or restore it to the War Department.

✠ T. Grant,
Bishop of Southwark.

My dear Rev. Mother,

The enclosed letters show that our decision regarding the expediency of receiving the *Sultan's* gift was founded on a false presumption. It seems now that the money is for the poor, that the Sisters are to be the almoners, and that their heroic charity has been the occasion or cause for selecting them to distribute amongst the poor the bounty of His Sublime Majesty of Constantinople.

Would it not appear, then, that there is no compromise of either feeling or principle in accepting the donations for distribution amongst the distressed? You can let me know your views, dear Rev. Mother, and return the letters, that I may send them back.—Yours sincerely,

✠ James Walsh.

The *Sultan's* gift was £230, divided between the different Communities that sent out Sisters.

We received innumerable letters from the poor soldiers, and I cannot close without giving a sample of one or two:

> I thank you kindly for all your goodness to me. I hope your reward is in store in Heaven for you and the remainder of your dear Sisters that served God, and with His help saved many a poor soldiers life.
> When far from a friend in a distant land, our meek Sisters brought the heavenly smile and the spirit of God into the wards among the broken-hearted soldiers. I can never forget your kindness. The Lord reward you for all your goodness and kindness to me! No more at present; but I remain, your faithful servant,
>
> Corporal James Brazil.

The following letter was written from Scutari, and forwarded to us at Balaklava:

> Dear Sister,
> I write to send my best respects to you, hoping they will be acceptable. For me to draw any inference from how very good and civil you were to me, is to think you won't be vexed with my audacity in enclosing a note for you. But if it displeases you, all you have to do is to tell Tom Connors that I should not enclose a note for you, and you will be obeyed. Dear Sister, the sergeant of the Rifles and myself unite in sending our best respects to you. Our feelings on this point are incomprehensible, we cannot express how lonesome we are since you left. Please do us the honour to write to us, dear Sister.—I have the honour to be
>
> Your obedient, humble servant,
>
> John Hopkins.

Appendix

Of the other group—the mainly English group—of Sisters of Mercy who worked quite separately from the mainly Irish group in the Crimea, a brief history should be made.

When the war between Russia and the Allied Armies of England and France broke out in 1854, and our Government resolved to send to the Crimea a regularly organised staff of nurses, of which Miss Florence Nightingale was placed at the head, Bishop Grant of Southwark obtained permission at once to place upon it a number of Sisters of Mercy. There was, however, at that time, but one Community of nuns in the Diocese of Southwark, within the limits of whose rules and vocation an undertaking of this sort seemed to lie.

The members of this Community were few in number, and were already fully occupied by their labours of love amongst the poor and sick in their own neighbourhood. Yet, when the bishop arrived one evening at their Convent in Bermondsey, and explained to the Superior the sad state of affairs, and dwelt on the terrible sufferings of the wounded soldiers, and on their need of good nursing, sisterly sympathy, and religious consolation, she offered herself and four other Sisters for the perilous mission.

Two days later the bishop wrote to the Superior to say that the Government wished them to go immediately—in fact, they were to start the very next morning. They had, therefore, only a few hours in which to prepare for a long and dangerous journey, with the details of which they were quite unacquainted, only knowing that they were to start for Turkey at half-past seven in the morning, and that they went for the love of God.

"And who is to take care of you from this to Turkey?" asked one of their amazed well-wishers. To which the Sisters only replied that "they hoped their angel guardians would kindly do so." Father Collingridge ran out and purchased for each Sister a railway rug and a small travelling bag, into which she stowed her clothes and books of devotion. Bishop Grant came the next morning, before the time of departure, to bid the travellers an affectionate goodbye. He gave them a letter of introduction to Mr. Goldsmid, a friend in Paris, which was their first halting-place, and recommended them to put up for the night at the *Hotel Meurice.*

On their arrival very late in the capital, they found the hotel full, and in their perplexity carried their letter to the house of Mr. Goldsmid. They were told that he had retired for the night, and nothing would induce his man-servant to disturb him. Tired with their journey, alone and friendless in a great city, they had a sense of desolation that was very acute. The servant, compassionating their plight, conducted them to the *Hotel Clarendon*, where, fortunately, they could be taken in, and were comfortably entertained.

Early the next morning Mr. Goldsmid arrived, bringing a telegram from Dr. Grant, desiring the Sisters to wait in Paris for a day or two, until further arrangements had been made. The Government having consented to ten nuns being placed on the staff of nurses, the bishop was most anxious to obtain five others to join those who had already started from Bermondsey. With this desire uppermost in his mind, he went to the Convent of the Faithful Virgin, at Norwood, to ask the orphans to pray for the additional volunteers.

"Here is permission to send ten nuns," he said to the Superior, "and I have only five."

"My Lord, she replied, after a thoughtful pause, "we have no mission for the service of the sick, but you can dispose of us as you think fit."

"God be praised!" said the bishop, and it was decided that on Monday morning—it being then Saturday—a party of five should be ready to start. There was a generous rivalry among the Sisters as to whom should be chosen for the difficult service; and when the five were duly selected they went at once into the chapel, and kneeling before our dear Lord in the Blessed Sacrament, they offered their lives to Him. Before six on Monday morning the bishop was at the station to bid them God-speed on their journey of love and self-sacrifice; but at the last parting his heart was too full to speak—he could only silently bless them.

The two detachments of nuns met in Paris, and, joining Miss Nightingale, they sailed together from Marseilles, and, after a rough voyage, in which the vessel was nearly lost, reached Scutari. On landing they were escorted by soldiers to the huge barracks, capable of holding five thousand men, which had been handed over for the use of the English by the *Sultan*, along with the adjoining hospital, containing accommodation for two thousand beds.

Nothing could be more desolate than the room allotted to the Sisters. Its only article of furniture was a decrepit chair; no fire could be obtained, and an icy wind blew through the broken windows. The luxury of a cup of tea, made with slightly warm water, and without milk or sugar, was obtained through the energy of a soldier; and this, along with a small slice of bread, constituted their first meal after landing on a foreign shore, worn out by the fatigue and sickness of the voyage.

The Battle of Inkerman was fought on the day following the arrival of the nurses, and henceforth the hospitals were crowded with the dying and the dead. How many lives were saved by the gentle ministrations of the Sisters those who were present at these awful scenes could, perhaps, form some idea; but how many souls gained eternally by the suggestions of faith and charity and contrition that fell from their lips on dying ears, will not be known until the day when those who bring many to righteousness shall shine with a sevenfold radiancy in the firmament of God.

Miss Grace Ramsay, from whose beautiful memoir of Bishop Grant we have gathered the facts here related, says:

> No painting, however graphic, could convey a true idea of what they, one and all, endured in their self-imposed warfare with death and sickness. In the stinging cold of an Eastern winter, when everything froze hard, they were without a fire; their food was scanty, and so bad that it reduced them to a choice between sickness and hunger. During the first six weeks of their arrival a drink of pure water was a luxury not to be had!

The Sisters had no second habits, so that when they came home, as they often did, drenched with rain, they had to remain in bed until the wet clothes were dried at the kitchen fire.

The soldiers vied with each other in paying attention to the Sisters. one of them writes from the Scutari barracks;

> You would be surprised at the nice feeling the men show, they are so cautious in their manners, and never utter a bad word or an oath before us. If one chances to say what the others think too free in our presence, the whole ward cry out 'hush!'

Still, the position of the Sisters was a trying one in the midst of three thousand soldiers; frequently coming into contact with foreigners, amongst others the Turks, who accosted them, respectfully enough, by the familiar name of "Johnny"; and, worse than all, deprived of all chance of solitude or of opportunities to join together in the performance of their habitual devotions. Very practical and very real were the every-day struggles of that life of charity and toil. Yet, on the other hand, as the writer before quoted observes:

> A poem undoubtedly it was, mystic and wonderful, but not visible in its beauty to common eyes. It was a poem attuned to no earthly key, but to the voice of souls enamoured of the Cross.

This heavenly music found an echo in the soul of Dr. Grant, who snatched time from his already well-filled hours to keep up a regular correspondence with his absent and "dear daughters in Christ," giving them all the home news, ever sympathising with them in their trials, and urging them to a close and closer union with their Divine Master, whose Passion he implores them ever to bear in mind. He tells them that even amid the hurry and noise of the wards they should be united to "the interior and mysterious life of their crucified Lord, and that their duties are only means to express their love for Him!" He urges them to "bear courageously all toil and suffering for the love of our sweet Lord, and to make amends for so many sinners who deny Him." He says:

> The best way to avoid distractions will be to recollect as often as possible that Christ, our dear Lord, lives in each of your sick flock; and so you will feel yourselves living in the immediate presence of Him Who has said: *'Whatever you do to one of these little ones is done to Me.'*

As time advances, and the winter is succeeded by an intensely hot summer, the bishop tells them that when overcome by the heat they must:

> Think of our dear Lord going about the same Asia, healing the sick, and obliged to rest at the well, and asking the Samaritan to give Him to drink.

At one time the bishop was greatly disturbed by rumours about an attempt to prevent the Sisters from speaking on matters of religion even to those of their own creed. He had written to them on their first setting out:

> Do not introduce religion to any but Catholics. When you can, suggest an act to the dying of contrition, faith, etc.

They had gone out, as he constantly reminds them, as nuns first and then nurses; and now, when he hears of a plan which is to reduce them to be nurses only, he writes to the Sisters to say that "it will be contrary to the express agreement with Government," and that if carried out, which fortunately it never was, their duty will plainly be to return home. Then, again, people said that the nuns did not work well with Miss Nightingale, and an ultra Protestant pamphlet appeared, pointing out the absurdity of "Catholic Nuns transferring their allegiance from the Pope of Rome to a Protestant lady." The tidings of these sayings and doings, when they reached Scutari, caused much merriment among the parties most nearly concerned. One of the Sisters playfully addressed Miss Nightingale as "Your Holiness," and the latter retorted by dubbing her "the Cardinal."

A year had now elapsed since the valiant little band had set out towards the East. Writes one in a letter home:

> What a dream, it all seems! One can scarcely believe that it will be a whole year next Wednesday since we left dear old Bermondsey. Yesterday there were great rejoicings for something—a victory gained, we know not where, for we live happily ignorant of all that goes on beyond the walls.

In the following month, for the second time, the cholera broke out at Scutari. The angel of death was indeed abroad, and many of the occupants of the hospital wards fell beneath the shadow of his wings. Two of the Sisters had been seriously ill for some time, but had stuck to their posts through all; and now a devoted lay-sister fell a victim to the raging epidemic, and was buried by the soldiers with every mark of affection and respect. Miss Nightingale was at Balaklava at the time, and she wrote to the Rev. Mother at Scutari, asking her, if possible, to get additional nuns from England. She concludes her letter thus:

> I cannot express to you, dear Rev. Mother, the gratitude which I and the whole country feel to you for your goodness. You have been one of our chief mainstays, and without you I do not know what would have become of the work. With love to all my Sisters, believe me, dear Rev. Mother, ever yours affectionately and gratefully, Florence Nightingale.

Consequently, three more Sisters found their way from Bermondsey to Scutari, though not in time to join in the Mass celebrated on the Christmas Day of 1855 by Father Bagshawe in the little chapel which had been appropriately decorated by the soldiers for the great festival. As Lent came on, the rigour of the climate and the continued strain and fatigue began to tell seriously on the health of the Sisters, and especially on that of the Rev. Mother. Bishop Grant writes, therefore, to beg them not to tax their strength further by fasting reminding them, by the way, that "Our dear Lord wishes us to look cheerful in Lent."

On Good Friday three of the Sisters accompanied Miss Nightingale to the "Front," and did service about five miles from Balaklava. They had a tent to themselves," we are told, "open to the weather in many parts, and on awaking next morning they found themselves covered with snow, which had fallen heavily all night. They were consoled for those little discomforts by the arrival of a gentleman on horseback bearing them the princely present of some eggs, tied up in a handkerchief.

The benefactor proved to be the Protestant chaplain of the detachment, who showed the nuns many other acts of kindness and courtesy, which they strove to acknowledge by washing his neckties, a process performed under difficulties, the teapot filled with boiling water doing duty as a smoothing iron. Miss Nightingale, writing from the new encampment to the Sisters at Scutari, says:

> I want my Cardinal very much up here. The Sisters are all quite well and cheerful, thank God for it! They have made their hut look quite tidy, and put up with the cold and inconveniences with the utmost self-abnegation. Everything, even the ink, freezes in our hut every night."

She writes again:

> Sister A—— is such a very steady worker, she has seven sick huts. Sister C—— is very commanding and courageous, and not easily daunted.

One of the nuns had a dangerous attack of fever, through which Miss Nightingale insisted on nursing her herself. One night, while watching by the sick-bed, she saw a huge rat upon the rafters right over the Sister's head; and taking an umbrella, she knocked it down and killed it without disturbing the patient.

And now at last, in April 1856, a peace was concluded; but, as the work among the wounded did not cease simultaneously with the cessation of the war, the Sisters still continued their stay in the East, with the exception of the Rev. Mother, whose shattered health and home duties rendered her return to England an imperative necessity "Work away merrily!" were her parting words to those whom she left behind at Balaklava and Scutari. In a farewell letter addressed to her by Florence Nightingale the latter says:

> You know that I shall do everything I can for the Sisters whom you have left me. I will care for them as if they were my own children. But it will not be like you. I do not presume to express praise or gratitude to you, Rev. Mother, because it would look as though I thought you had done this work, not unto God, but unto me. You were far above me in fitness for the general superintendency in worldly talent of administration, and far more in the spiritual qualifications which God values in a Superior; my being placed over you was my misfortune, not my fault. What you have done for the work no one can ever say. I do not presume to give you any other tribute but my tears. But I should be glad that the Bishop of Southwark should know, and Dr. Manning, that you were valued here as you deserve, and that the gratitude of the army is yours.

The other Sisters remained more than two months longer on the scene of their long and loving labours; their return to England being commemorated by Bishop Grant in a Pastoral, in which he spoke of them as those who had "earned for themselves not, indeed, the perishable glory of earthly victory, but the promise of everlasting reward and of unfading crowns."

The Sisters had from the first refused all remuneration for their services; and when, after their return to England, Lord Panmure wrote to:

> Express to the Sisterhood the sense entertained by Her Majesty's Government of the devotion displayed by them in attending the sick and wounded soldiers in the British hospitals in the East,

And to offer them a sum of money, the nuns generously declined it, expressing at the same time a willingness, which the Government readily gratified, to distribute it among the poor and sick of their own district, preferring for themselves to be rewarded only by His grace and love, for whose sake alone they had undertaken a difficult and a noble work.

****

The following correspondence has in this very Jubilee Year, 1897, passed between the queen, and the author of this volume:

Pall Mall, London, S.W.,
February 15th, 1897.

Madam,

The Queen having been pleased to bestow upon you the decoration of the Royal Red Cross, I have to inform you that in the case of such honours as this it is the custom of Her Majesty to personally bestow the decoration upon the recipient when such a course is convenient to all concerned , and I have, therefore, to request that you will be so good as to inform me whether it would be convenient to you to attend at Windsor sometime within the next few weeks. Should any circumstances prevent your receiving the Royal Red Cross from the hands of Her Majesty, it could be transmitted by post to your present address.

I am, Madam, your obedient servant,

George M. Farquharson.

Sister Mary Aloysius.

St. Patrick's, Gort, county Galway
February 17th, 1897.

Sir,

I received your letter of the 15th, intimating to me that Her Most Gracious Majesty the Queen is pleased to bestow on me the Order of the Royal Cross, in recognition of the services of my Sisters in religion and my own in caring for the wounded soldiers at the Crimea during the war. My words cannot express my gratitude for the great honour which Her Majesty is pleased to confer upon me. The favour is, if possible, enhanced by the permission to receive this public mark of favour at Her Majesty's own hands. The weight of seventy-six years and the infirmities of age will, I trust, dispense me from the journey to the Palace. I will, therefore, with sentiments of deepest gratitude, ask to be permitted to receive this mark of my Sovereign's favour in the less public and formal manner you have kindly indicated.

I am, Sir,
Faithfully yours in Jesus Christ,
Sister M. Aloysius,

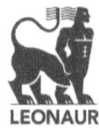

ALSO FROM LEONAUR
AVAILABLE IN SOFTCOVER OR HARDCOVER WITH DUST JACKET

THE WOMAN IN BATTLE by Loreta Janeta Velazquez—Soldier, Spy and Secret Service Agent for the Confederacy During the American Civil War.

BOOTS AND SADDLES by Elizabeth B. Custer—The experiences of General Custer's Wife on the Western Plains.

FANNIE BEERS' CIVIL WAR by Fannie A. Beers—A Confederate Lady's Experiences of Nursing During the Campaigns & Battles of the American Civil War.

LADY SALE'S AFGHANISTAN by Florentia Sale—An Indomitable Victorian Lady's Account of the Retreat from Kabul During the First Afghan War.

THE TWO WARS OF MRS DUBERLY by Frances Isabella Duberly—An Intrepid Victorian Lady's Experience of the Crimea and Indian Mutiny.

THE REBELLIOUS DUCHESS by Paul F. S. Dermoncourt—The Adventures of the Duchess of Berri and Her Attempt to Overthrow French Monarchy.

LADIES OF WATERLOO by Charlotte A. Eaton, Magdalene de Lancey & Juana Smith—The Experiences of Three Women During the Campaign of 1815: Waterloo Days by Charlotte A. Eaton, A Week at Waterloo by Magdalene de Lancey & Juana's Story by Juana Smith.

NURSE AND SPY IN THE UNION ARMY by Sarah Emma Evelyn Edmonds—During the American Civil War

WIFE NO. 19 by Ann Eliza Young—The Life & Ordeals of a Mormon Woman During the 19th Century

DIARY OF A NURSE IN SOUTH AFRICA by Alice Bron—With the Dutch-Belgian Red Cross During the Boer War

MARIE ANTOINETTE AND THE DOWNFALL OF ROYALTY by Imbert de Saint-Amand—The Queen of France and the French Revolution

THE MEMSAHIB & THE MUTINY by R. M. Coopland—An English lady's ordeals in Gwalior and Agra duringthe Indian Mutiny 1857

MY CAPTIVITY AMONG THE SIOUX INDIANS by Fanny Kelly—The ordeal of a pioneer woman crossing the Western Plains in 1864

WITH MAXIMILIAN IN MEXICO by Sara Yorke Stevenson—A Lady's experience of the French Adventure

AVAILABLE ONLINE AT **www.leonaur.com**
AND FROM ALL GOOD BOOK STORES

www.ingramcontent.com/pod-product-compliance
Lightning Source LLC
Chambersburg PA
CBHW031621160426
43196CB00006B/221